Verity Craig is a magazine editor, former magazine owner and current business owner of two restaurants, along with her husband, Paul.

Before embarking on her magazine editorship career, she was a freelance writer for magazines, followed by chief writer and sub-editor, working in-house for local publications.

This is Verity's first book.

"Never judge a man until you have walked a mile in his moccasins."

Native American Proverb

To those of you reading this who are going through infertility, I've walked in your shoes, I know your pain. This book is for you.
Dedicated to Niomi and Daisy-May.

Verity Craig

IVF and Infertility, Our Journey: A True Story of One Couple's Struggle Against the Odds

AUSTIN MACAULEY PUBLISHERS™
LONDON • CAMBRIDGE • NEW YORK • SHARJAH

A CIP catalogue record for this title is available from the British Library.

ISBN 9781788786485 (Paperback)
ISBN 9781788786492 (E-Book)

www.austinmacauley.com

First Published (2018)
Austin Macauley Publishers Ltd™
25 Canada Square
Canary Wharf
London
E14 5LQ

Acknowledgements

Writing this book has been a journey. Reading through the events in my diary that Paul and I were faced with has trawled up many emotional memories that I had subconsciously pushed to the back of my mind. In many ways, it has been a Pandora's box of memoirs from one of the most difficult stages in our lives.

But with it also came reminders of who was there for Paul and me at what was the most traumatic period of our life together.

Firstly, I'd like to acknowledge both of our families, especially all of our parents (I say 'all' because we have the most wonderful step-parents too), for their understanding of the pain that we went through while also being so supportive and for simply letting us know they were there whenever we needed them. We probably can't fully appreciate how difficult it must have been for you watching us from the wings and hoping it would be a happy ending for us, while at the same time, you were also longing for that new little addition in the family, too. Thank you.

To my mother, the walks around the park to talk and those chats over cups of tea with cake really helped clear my mind, remain positive and focus again. Thank you, too, for coming to a couple of those doctor's meetings with me. It must have all been very hard for you to hear, too.

Niomi, my daughter, thank you for your understanding and being patient through all of this journey. I can only imagine that there were times when it must have also been so difficult for you to witness. In many ways, it's your doing that we wanted a baby so desperately; you really have always been the perfect daughter to me, I am so very blessed. Your encouragement with this book from its beginning has meant so much to me, too.

At times like this, one should never underestimate their friends. We decided to keep our journey as private as possible, but there were a few dear friends whom we did confide in. Lauren Johns, you know most of this story without reading the book! Thank you for all those lunches where we would mull it over, you would support me and let me talk (and somehow we would laugh and you always made me depart feeling happy again). All women need friends like you.

Paula Seabourne-Pearson, what can I say? Thank you for just understanding that we were going through something traumatic. Those simple nods and winks at business events or social parties just to check that I was OK meant so much and won't ever be forgotten. I will always treasure you, my dear friend.

Barbara Mishon, thank you 'Aunty Barbara', for always believing in us. Through all that you were also going through in your life at that time, you still kept telling us 'it will happen'. I still have that newspaper-cutting in my desk drawer that you posted to me about an article claiming that 'raspberries could help with infertility'. All of your care and love means so much (Jessie and James, you too)!

Helen Shenston, your healing hands on me trying to aid something to happen, and simply your kind words, meant so much to me, especially after a couple of traumatic times we went through in particular. You know what I mean. Thank you.

Mo Hunter-Shine, I always said you were 'my rock' at the magazine, didn't I? And I discovered that it extended into our friendship when I confided in you some of what we were going through. I was so lucky that you were my right-hand person at that period in my working life but even luckier to have gained you as a friend.

Peter James, as an acclaimed author, your advice has been of the most superior knowledge that I could have ever wished for. You took me under your experienced wing with guidance while also having such faith in me about writing this book, even when I didn't. In addition, your friendship and understanding of what Paul and I went through was second to none. Thank you also for passing me over to the wonderful Susan Opie.

Susan, thank you for casting your experienced eyes over my book when it was simply a manuscript that had only been proofed by a couple of close family members.

Michael Dooley, it was fate in the form of your book that brought us together, so thank goodness for literature! Your intellectual knowledge on infertility and IVF, with your down-to-earth attitude, kept us going. You told us the facts and scientific know-how, and at the same time, you were always there for us, however busy you were. Sorry if we bombarded you with texts and emails! Thank you for always replying. In addition, I must say a very emotional thank you to you for actually saving my life. At a time when I did not suspect anything wrong, over the phone, you advised me to get help at a critical time. You also put us in touch with a place that would change our journey forever, The Lister Hospital.

Where do I begin with The Lister Hospital? So many people there to thank, who, over the years, also became our friends. Sonographers Jhalia, Liz and Alison, thank you for your support and kind words of understanding at such a horrible time over and over again when we were sat with you in anticipation, looking at the screen. Alison, thank you for caring for me when you had to break some terrible news to me. Sorry we put you through that. On happier times, we enjoyed chatting with you over the years about your cats!

Safira Bartha, who heads up the embryologist department at The Lister, from when you first visited us upon hearing that there was a concerned couple in reception about a front-page newspaper article they had seen on IVF, we liked and connected with you instantly. Professional and calm, you explained in great detail to us why this article was misleading on so many levels. After that, you took the time to call us and visit us whenever we were at The Lister to check how we were doing. You are a very special person who we will always treasure for the way that you looked after us. Sorry for making you work so extra hard on that microscope! We also thank your lovely team of embryologists, as well as the nurses and the doctors.

Dr Marie Wren, thank you, especially for your caring sympathy when there were tears.

And Raef Faris, well, how do you say thank you to someone that has done so much for you over and above what is expected of them professionally, who has also become a friend? Your kindness, but also professionalism, throughout was both noble and generous. However busy you were (and I know you were), you always texted or called me back immediately. And whenever we doubted ourselves, you would pick us up again. Your spiritual nature, mixed with your medical expertise, is the perfect making for a doctor working in your field. We are fortunate to have found you and to have gained a friend. Thank you also for your support and enthusiasm in me creating this book. You said it is a much-needed tool for infertility patients. I do hope you are right and that we do help even one couple.

I'd also like to thank anyone else who offered us kind words of support and also showed me support in producing this book.

And finally, my husband, Paul. Wow, what a journey, hey! It's clichéd, but I love you, and thank you for simply being there. I'm sorry for us that we had to endure the experience that we did, but we don't believe in regrets, do we? Thank you for just holding my hand when I needed it and for being so very brave; I know how tough it's been for you too. You've shown me what true strength is and I will always admire that in you. Thank you for also helping me make this dream of a book a reality. Whenever I doubted it would happen, you would quickly get me into shape like a coach with your forthwith manner and off I'd go to add a few more bits that we had remembered. Without you, this book certainly would not have happened.

I'd also like to say an additional and sincere thank you to you, the readers, for simply reading this book. For those of you that need it, I truly do hope that it helps you in some manner. And together, let's break down the taboo shroud that surrounds infertility.

For those of you that know people going through infertility, I hope this book assists you a little bit in supporting and understanding them a bit more.

And to Daisy-May…you were worth every single hour, minute and second of waiting. Never could we use the word 'miracle' to describe anything more worthy than you.

Foreword written by Consultant Gynaecologist, Mr Michael Dooley MMS FFSRH FRCOG, who consults at a handful of highly-respected hospitals and is author of *Fit for Fertility*.

It is with great pleasure to provide a foreword to *IVF and Infertility, Our Journey*, written by Verity Craig.

Planning a baby, experiencing problems and undergoing tests and treatment is not only just about medical issues, it does have a huge emotional, as well as a financial burden, which is often under estimated. It is so important that this issue is discussed and shared.

Verity has done this in an exceptionally well written and informative book. The rollercoaster of a journey that Verity and Paul went through is not only fascinating but also heart breaking. Their commitment to this journey was unbelievable and their honest appraisal of the infertility 'business' an eye opener. It is always an honour and privilege to be involved in a fertility journey, but to be able to read this diary and be able to get some understanding of the significant ups and downs is so important to me, as a doctor, with over 30 years' experience in the fertility world.

The management of a couple undergoing fertility treatment is true teamwork and this book should be read by all the team involved in care. It will give them an in-depth understanding of the often very rough seas that the couple have to endure.

Also, anyone undergoing fertility treatment should read it, to help them understand that they are not alone. A problem shared is a problem halved.

I really must congratulate Verity and Paul for their honesty and dedication and allowing us all to have an insight into their journey.

Daisy-May will be proud of them.

Verity, a big thank you from me for helping other patients.

Foreword written by Mr Raef Faris, MSc FRCOG
Consultant Gynaecologist at the Lister Hospital, Chelsea, London.

I have been Verity and Paul's consultant through their incredible fertility journey. It started with a consultation for a second opinion after several failed IVFs, but ended up with a friendship that I personally treasure.

Verity and Paul have been through numerous recurrent implantation failures which leaves a couple with many unanswered questions and uncertainty. In addition, they also suffered miscarriages, and then a ruptured ectopic which in addition of being a pregnancy loss in its entity, is also a serious medical emergency which needs urgent surgical intervention.

As their consultant gynaecologist, I have seen them pull through the unknown and unanswered questions, which is brilliantly illustrated in this book. It was never all doom and gloom as people may imagine. We had numerous meetings and phone calls and as tough as our meetings could often be, all three of us somehow always managed to joke and keep upbeat. Perhaps, that helped Paul and Verity to some extent. Each couple I meet has a different way of coping both in the clinic setting and their daily life. I believe that trying to sense the couple's mechanisms of handling their predicament is an important role of a fertility doctor. The need of factual information should also come hand in hand with humane understanding and empathy.

As I was reading this book, I could relate to it as their treating doctor bringing back memories that I treasure, but also as one who has had his own infertility journey.

I believe that this book has a rich and detailed description of emotional and physical constraints that came with this journey easily described in a natural way without any artificial make up or masks.

This book describes the details of Verity and Paul's journey in a depth blended with many aspects of their day-to-day life and how they pull through their ups and downs. It describes several factors and parameters that were affected and how they affected their journey.

This book describes a story that could put many life aspects to the test. There aren't many books that describe in very simple words the way in which couples present their viewpoints during their different phases of fertility treatment. As I was close to Verity and Paul during their treatment journey, I can see how this book tells their story first hand, honestly and unpolished.

Preface

Having experienced several years of 'unexplained infertility', my husband, Paul, and I were flung in to an often-unspoken world of pain and heartache when we struggled to have a baby together.

As well as the hundreds of hospital and clinic trips for advice, we wanted to seek advice at home. One way of seeking this information was by scrawling the Internet for books in the hope that they would provide us with some help and support in finding procedures that were available, but also of first hand emotional and personal experiences so that we would then know exactly what to expect. While there are thousands of books written by medical professionals on the subject, we could not find any books written by anyone actually going through infertility themselves.

With one in six couples experience infertility across the world, infertility is not uncommon; it affects all ethnic backgrounds, all classes and all ages. Fertility forums online are one of the biggest areas for chat rooms on the Internet. This is what encouraged me to start recording all of my notes as a diary during our difficult and often traumatic journey in the hope that one day I could transform my notes into a book to help other couples and individuals across the world. Being a magazine editor and journalist by trade, writing is also my natural outlet.

As a couple finding ourselves experiencing this harrowing time in our lives, we discovered that when we read online of other couples' advice or tips of what helped them either get pregnant or of just what supported them, it helped us emotionally hugely, while also loading us with ammunition of subjects to discuss with our doctors in forthcoming meetings. We are not a unique couple.

Infertility is a big subject, but also a big secret often brushed under the carpet; people feel ashamed and society often makes them feel that way. With this book, it is my hope that it might help tear down the taboo shroud that surrounds this problem that sadly affects so many. As an extremely private person myself, I must admit that right up until publishing this book, I have struggled with whether, on a personal note, I am doing the right thing. However, I keep coming back to this strong desire to help others by sharing our story, while also encouraging society to open up a little about this subject and be sympathetic.

In a world where we now discuss, debate or read of the most shocking subjects freely, for some reason struggling and longing to produce new life is still one of the biggest off-limits subjects of all.

Being as common problem as it is, behind the scenes the fertility world is a big business.

So, it is my hope that this book not only demonstrates the emotional upheaval that this unexpected journey can entail upon people, but also the financial impact as well as how to avoid the sharks that are out there offering 'to get you pregnant'. It's very sad, but while being in this emotional state, you will want to literally try anything that could help, and there are some not-so-very-nice people out there knowing this that are ready to prey on you with potions, notions and unproven advice, so be cautious.

However, where there is darkness there is light. And so thankfully there are some amazingly kind and gifted individuals and clinics that can offer sincere professional help, and I mention them in this book. It is my aim to tell you our whole story, from all the negative experiences right through to the people, clinics and procedures that helped us and may also help you. Obviously, every situation is different. However, there may be one little piece of the jigsaw that you haven't yet tried and don't yet know about, that may just fit for you. I don't want to say 'work' because at the end of the day, as much as we try, we are all still in the hands of the gods so to speak – fate. I would hate to ever imply that what works for one person, would definitely work for another.

Finally, this book is written from the heart with honesty about our struggle with infertility and IVF. It has been deliberately written in colloquial diary format to make it simple for you, the reader, to easily visit and re-visit different fertility cycles or date lines that may be appropriate for you.

I must warn you that our journey through infertility is one of quite shocking consequences time and time again. This could not have been predicted when I commenced writing this book, and I hope it does not deter you from continuing to try. From clinics where the experience was distressing and unprofessional to life-threatening experiences, our story is one of high peaks and lows. However, it is a real and truthful journey that I hope will spur you on, and if it can help support just one couple out there reading this, then I have achieved exactly what I set out to do. I would love to hear from you too.

Finally, if you are experiencing infertility, take a breath, stay positive and find your inner strength – everyone has it.

You can email Verity direct on: info@chocolateboxpublishing.com

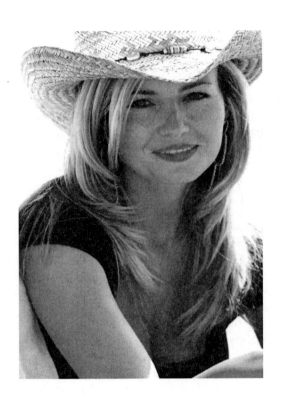

An Introduction to Us

Many years ago, I watched a television documentary presented by the pioneering doctor, Professor Robert Winston, where the viewer followed couples he was treating for infertility. It was the UK's first fly-on-the-wall introduction to the traumatic but ground-breaking world of IVF. It was also a celebration of this revolutionary technique in our modern world.

At the time of watching this, I already had my beautiful daughter, Niomi; my surprise baby from when I was 17 years old, who changed my life forever in a great and wonderful way, despite my having her so young.

I remember thinking back then as I watched these brave couples' individual journeys, what terrible pain they must be feeling and how it must be so hard to keep going against the odds; to keep hope alive after all their setbacks.

One couple in the programme stood out in my mind, and still does today. The lady already had a child from a previous relationship. The man did not. I expect that I and other viewers could correctly be accused of *initially* not being as sympathetic to them as to the other couples, since the lady was already a mother and, likewise, the husband a stepfather.

However, I recall that as the series progressed it became clear just how terrible what they were going through was for this couple; and how incredibly brave they were, longing for a child together.

So it was deeply ironic that I (and many others I'm sure) ended up feeling such immense sympathy for this poor couple in particular.

The heartache that we, the viewers, witnessed of this husband and wife (and the other couples) who clearly had such a great love for one another, was heart breaking. It always stayed with me.

In my own world, I can remember at the time continually thinking that my wonderful daughter was given to me at a young age for a reason; always counting my blessings. People would ask me then, and still do, how did you cope with a baby so young? Maybe the fact that I subsequently managed to forge what was recognised as a successful career while being a single mother made it more surprising (I'd owned a business and subsequently became a journalist and editor). My answer has always been the same; given any situation in life, you just cope, don't you? Go in to autopilot and do your very best; that is exactly what I did. But above all, I loved this little being with all my heart in a way that nothing could compete! Looking back now, I just hope I did 'OK'. I also had my wonderful mother's support in particular. And in any case, I always say that people go through far tougher experiences in life. My daughter was a blessing after all. I can't even imagine life without her. As clichéd as it may sound, she has always been my everything, and I cherish that.

Forward wind quite a few years, upon meeting my husband-to-be (and love of my life) at the apparently sensible adult age of 29, I thought I could finally be what is perceived as a 'normal-aged' mum. When I met Paul, my daughter Niomi was 11 years old. Paul was 34.

There was immense love between us immediately. I can remember saying naïvely to my mother soon after meeting him, "He is such a nice guy! I can see us being great friends." And what better base is there for a relationship than friendship? I wasn't the sort of girl to do the 'dating circuit'. That world just wasn't me. So I guess it hadn't dawned on me at that moment that I had actually met 'the one'. Friends always said to me, "The one will come along when you least expect it." So right were they!

At that time, I had managed to work my way up quickly in my career from being a freelance journalist to a chief writer for a magazine to then being invited to be the editor of a magazine that the same publishing company I worked for had purchased. The purchase was big news at this particular publishing house and also in my hometown, and a lot of people were interviewed for the position, so I was thrilled at this career opportunity, and I absolutely loved it. Meanwhile, Paul, who already owned numerous businesses, opened a new restaurant/bar that the 'it' crowd of our hometown were flooding to (from Hollywood actress Joan Collins to television presenter Zoe Ball and their friends).

My daughter, Niomi, was thriving at school too, gaining a music scholarship, later transferred to an academic one. And most of all, she was happy. It was a fun and joyful time. Then, Paul and I fulfilled a business vision I had had for many years; to create our own lifestyle magazine. With Paul's business acumen and my editorial background and business contacts, we launched a local high-end lifestyle glossy magazine; its success beat all of our expectations. It was a gamble, but boy did it work. We subsequently launched it in London. I guess, naïvely at that time, we felt like an invincible couple; but we always appreciated that we were lucky and had both in our separate ways worked very hard and honestly to carve our careers from a young age.

I started to be able to grab the odd night out with Paul, making up for all those years of being a young, single mum who was in rather a lot.

Just after the exciting and successful launch of our new business venture together, our magazine, we went away to Barbados (we had booked it in advance or there's no way we would have so soon after launching)! On a beautiful evening on white sands lying on our own with the warm sea lapping gently around us by sunset, Paul amazed and thrilled me by proposing. Our dreams were all coming true. We were truly blessed. And untouchable.

So, two years later in August 2008, having known since we first met we wanted to have children together (and give Niomi siblings), we thought I should come off of the contraceptive pill a month prior to our wedding. So sure were we I would fall pregnant quickly, I can remember us discussing at the time, "Imagine if I fall pregnant straightaway and suffer morning sickness during our wedding!" Little did we know back then what we know now. How 'happy go lucky' were we!

Well, now my husband, Paul, and I are *that* couple that I watched all those years ago in that documentary series, the couple who always stayed in my mind. And this is our incredible fertility story...

My Fertility Diary...

November 2009:

It's been a stressful year and a half of us being introduced to the world of infertility. To begin with, my GP assured me that despite me not becoming pregnant for a year, we had 'nothing to worry about'. And with all the necessary tests on both Paul and I coming back as 'normal', we believed that to be the case.

However, still nothing happened...for several more months.

I have now invested financially and emotionally in so-called fertility acupuncture, massage, various special diets (which include living on such things as green tea, pineapple and almonds, while completely cutting out caffeine and sugar), but so far my efforts have been in vain. It's a hopeless feeling. It's horrible not being able to control it.

We have hope day in day out that it may happen, but still nothing. It's awful and scary not knowing what the future will hold in this area of our lives. We are being told 'it will happen if you just relax', but all we can do is worry. And every month when that period of mine rears its ugly head, we both sigh in sadness. Meanwhile, every pregnancy test we do if I am a day or two late, flashes back at us blatantly 'not pregnant'.

I think that because I fell pregnant with my daughter, Niomi, in such a sudden unexpected way, I always expected I would again. How stupid was I? Meanwhile, close people to us that know we are trying for a baby echo my doctor's words by telling me to relax and that it will then happen. But it's not as though I am uptight about it, and I do understand what they mean. But it's been nearly two years of trying for a baby now and I can't help but feel anxious. Also, now at 35 years old, I'm very aware of my age making it harder to fall pregnant...the clock ticking like this is enough to make anyone feel the pressure.

Anyway, we recently visited a local fertility clinic in Hove, which turned out to be a daunting episode and terrible mistake. In fact, a disaster.

Having read in my own magazine about how amazing, compassionate and professional this clinic on our doorstep apparently was, it seemed the obvious place for us to try as our first port of call. I of all people should know to never believe the advertorials you read in magazines! But when you're in the infertility world, you jump at anything that says it could 'help you on your journey to having a baby'.

Our initial meeting with the doctor who owned it, was very official and cold. When you're in this situation, it's a very lonely place; all you want is some compassion when you do open up and discuss it. We were told in a very matter-of-fact way which blood tests we would need to have at this stage (many were repeats of the ones my GP had already done, only this time we had to pay…a lot. But she insisted we need to have them done again), and we were also told that they didn't carry out any procedures, such as IVF, on their premises; if we required them, we would have to have them at our local NHS hospital. And yet, we would have to pay for it since the NHS would not allow us to have any IVF cycles through them as I already had a daughter.

Incidentally, if you are single, foreign or a same sex couple you are entitled to two or three cycles on the NHS in England, and rightfully so.

However, what I find frustrating is that the NHS is so averse to single parents re-marrying and starting a family again. I find this especially cruel if their new partner is childless, as in our case. Surely, in a land where people are receiving plastic surgery for vanity purposes on the NHS nowadays, anyone should be entitled to at least one IVF cycle? Fortunately, at this stage, we can pay for our treatment. However, I think it is so desperately sad for couples who find themselves in the same situation as us but cannot afford the extortionate cost.

Anyway, we are embarking upon more tests. As with anything that will give us an insight as to why I'm not falling pregnant right now, we agreed to have the tests (again) at the clinic and awaited the results; since we had already had most of these we felt confident that they should all be fine and so we didn't think much more of it.

A week or two later, I received a phone call from the fertility clinic asking me to come in. I informed them that my husband was in London for work for the day and asked if it was urgent as I could call him to come with me. In a very nonchalant way, I was told it was 'nothing urgent or to worry about, and to just pop down' to see them.

I don't know why, maybe I had a feeling, but I asked my mother to come with me; me, who is usually so fiercely independent. And, thank goodness I did.

We waited in the open area in front of the reception desk (where everyone can hear you checking in, not private at all). I was called through nearly an hour after my booked appointment. I went in the room alone. The doctor got straight to the point in her usual manner, same as before. She informed me in a very serious but matter-of-act way with no compassion, that my blood test results were terrifyingly low (with an AMH level of 1), and that it was now 'impossible' that I would ever get pregnant.

In one instant, my whole world crashed down around me. How could this be? I have a daughter? I am only in my mid-30s. I'd been told from these previous test results that everything was fine. She went on to say that I was prematurely going in to the menopause. It got worse! There really was nothing good to say in fact. And all I wanted was for Paul to be with me. Then the doctor's mobile phone rang while she was informing me of this terrible news. To my amazement, she answered it and chatted about collecting someone; her child I remember guessing. It was a personal phone call. The real world, and hers, was carrying on around me while I was being given this devastating news. It was surreal. I was in shock at what was happening and I suddenly felt sick. I'd gone from being the girl who fell pregnant so easily at a young age, (to being careful from then on after) to now being told that I was infertile.

After a few minutes, I returned to the waiting room where my mother was. I just looked at her and said 'let's go' while trying not to crumble in to tears. I knew if I started, I wouldn't be able to stop.

When we reached the lift, that's when I suddenly burst in to uncontrollable tears and told her what I had just been informed; I had stomach-churning pain. My body ached from within. My mother was immediately furious at the clinic, as it became quickly clear that I had not been given any detailed information or explanation, and also that on the phone that day they had said it was not necessary for my husband to be with me. How much worse in the fertility world could it get than being told 'you'll never fall pregnant'?

Over the following weeks, I continued with the diets, massages and fertility acupuncture…and frantic internet trawling every day. I just felt, I couldn't stop everything and give up yet. My acupuncturist, Yvonne, who specialised in this area (I discovered her after seeing a story on television about her on our local BBC news, about helping women fall pregnant), was baffled by the results when I told her. She was convinced something was wrong with these results. I decided to get all of the tests repeated, at my GP's surgery again, and thankfully, he agreed.

Days later, to my amazement and confusion, the results came back as 'normal' for my age (AMH 7.9)! What on earth was going on? Why had the fertility clinic told me it was 1? With AMH, you can expect a slight change day to day, but not as dramatic as this. No one, not even my GP could understand it. I felt like I was tearing my hair out.

I called the fertility clinic to inform them what had happened. I was told by a nurse that the doctor would call me back to discuss this. They have never called me to this day.

However, what I did receive was a rather odd letter a few days after my phone call to them which stated that my results were now indeed almost identical to those from my GP (it said my AMH was 7). In the covering letter, there was no mention of my recent meeting with the doctor and no mention of the previous devastatingly low results that she had given me (for this same test). And certainly no apology or admission of what was clearly a terrible mistake on their part. We felt that the letter was to possibly cover themselves legally.

I now gather that my original results were in fact someone else's. That poor person who went from having my higher result, to their own.

Needless to say, we did not want to return to this clinic in Hove again.

Meanwhile, although I was not seeing a 'pregnancy' result from the acupuncture, I felt that it was really helping me emotionally and giving me strength physically; I also had that hopeful feeling that it might just help boost my fertility. The lovely lady, Yvonne, who carried out the acupuncture from her practice in Burgess Hill, gave me a book to read one week. This book would change everything for Paul and I, and lead the path to our fertility journey in a more positive way.

The book was called *Fit for Fertility*, and it was written by Michael Dooley.

Continuation of November 2009 to December 2009...

As soon as I started reading *Fit for Fertility*, I was hooked. I read pages and pages every day and night, and found myself reading poignant paragraphs that I could relate to, or that gave me hope, out loud to Paul. We were both sure that the author was someone we should talk to. His name was Dr Michael Dooley, a highly respected gynaecologist who specialised in infertility (and who we later discovered incidentally has worked for the Royal family).

I would strongly recommend to anyone going through infertility, they read this book. It discusses in detail scientific and holistic facts about what can affect couples' chances of becoming pregnant. I found it to be a really good insight to what this infertility world is all about.

Upon completing the book one evening, and feeling quite blown away by what I read and simply desperate, Paul and I decided to construct an email about our journey so far and a brief medical history to Dr Michael Dooley in the hope that he would see us for a consultation one day. His email address was in the back of the book. We were aware, however, that he must have been inundated by such desperate emails, so we thought if at all, a reply would take some time.

Within an hour, we received a reply from him personally inviting us to contact his secretary to arrange a meeting as soon as possible at his chambers in London at The King Edward VII's Hospital. We were both amazed and touched by his fast and personal response. He said how very sorry he was to read our email but felt sure he could help us in some way. Something felt good about it, and we were right. We went to sleep that night feeling slightly uplifted about our chances now for a change. Maybe this was someone who would want to help us at last.

We met with Michael two weeks later. He asked us each to bring an up to date medical history and details of how long we had been trying for a baby. We gave him everything and answered all of his questions as clearly as we could while he wrote it all down in front of us. He was very forthright that something more could be done immediately to help our situation and hopefully give us the baby that we both so longed for. He kept saying that we hadn't really tried many avenues yet and that there were lots of options available for us.

We left his office feeling positive for the first time in ages! We felt as though he was more on our level and far more professional and caring than our previous experience with a fertility doctor.

In front of us, he had dictated a letter for his secretary to write to The Lister Fertility Clinic that he worked with, which was based in The Lister Hospital, Chelsea.

He had explained to us that IVF was a good route to go down, but that first there were some other options that we should try at The Lister. I was relieved, as the idea of IVF terrified me. I always said to Paul that I didn't think I could ever do it. It was a real fear of mine. Maybe it was seeing those couples go through IVF all those years ago on that television documentary that had cemented a fear in me. Or maybe, it's simply because IVF has such a scary stigma attached to it for women. It's also stepping in to the unknown both emotionally and physically. The idea of injecting needles in to yourself daily, having internal scans and followed by a big procedure, knowing it's still only a gamble, is a frightening step to embark upon.

Paul and I were about to go away on a short holiday when Dr Michael Dooley suggested I see him beforehand so that we could plan the next step. Since it was a last minute appointment, Paul was already busy, and so my mother accompanied me as she was the only person who knew that we had now accepted one way or another, that we now needed medical intervention (and I wanted someone to take notes).

Michael discussed the drug Clomid and IUI (intrauterine insemination or artificial insemination) as options that we should initially consider trying. He explained that Clomid was a drug taken daily during the monthly cycle that basically boosted egg production thus increasing the chances of a pregnancy that month. IUI meanwhile was where drugs were injected in to the woman daily to boost egg production, and then at the time of ovulation the man's sperm sample was taken and 'washed' and then placed inside the woman through a speculum in the cervix or higher. IUI is usually only offered to women under 40 years of age as it carries less chance of working over that age. Apparently, it should feel the same as a pap smear with little or no discomfort. It was mostly the thought of the injections that I feared.

We also touched on the dreaded IVF subject. Michael Dooley summed it up perfectly for me when I asked how it is in comparison to going through IUI. He said, "An IUI is like a shandy, whereas IVF is more like a whisky!"

FACT BOX:

IUI: IUI stands for intrauterine insemination.

IUI is a form of assisted conception. During IUI, a doctor places washed, prepared sperm into the female uterus (womb) and near to their egg at their time of ovulation. This procedure is often combined with fertility drugs that are injected daily to increase chances of conceiving.

Clomid: Clomid (clomiphene) is a non-steroidal tablet-form fertility medicine.

It causes the pituitary gland to release hormones needed to stimulate ovulation (the release of an egg from the ovary).

Clomid is often used to cause ovulation in women who have been struggling to fall pregnant naturally.

Diary continues…4th January 2010:

So, over to The Lister Fertility Clinic it was.

The Lister is an impressive and clean hospital. The staff are all friendly and caring. And the environment is discreet; waiting areas are spread out and televisions are always switched on so there is none of that awkward nerve-wracking silence often found in such waiting rooms where couples find themselves whispering to one another. Someone at The Lister has clearly considered this.

Our visits to The Lister were not that frequent initially. We were again informed by one of the doctors there about Clomid.

The more we were hearing about Clomid, the more excited we became about it, for if it worked it would be a simple solution wonder drug. Naturally, we went home and read up on the internet all about it. It seemed to have worked for so many couples! We were excited.

Meanwhile, on a positive note, Paul was awarded Entrepreneur of The Year at the prestigious Sussex Business Awards. It was great to see how much it lifted him! We took Niomi, Paul's lovely parents and my father and his partner Janet. Paul had worked so hard all of his adult life so it was really thrilling to see it being recognised. As well as our joint publishing business together, Paul has also owned restaurant and cocktail bars over the years (of which I am now getting more and more involved in running with him). He started his oldest business, however, at the tender age of 16. It is a successful commercial sound, light, design and build company working mostly within the restaurant and bar industry. He is what the true meaning of the word 'entrepreneur' is (it's so often used in haste these days, in my opinion).

Paul's speech was very touching especially thanking his mother and stepfather, John, for all that they have done for him over the years supporting him tirelessly. They are amazing people. And me...yes, he thanked me too which was nice. It was a very emotional and thrilling evening.

It nearly didn't happen, however, as there was an unusually heavy downpour of snow that day. But the amazing organisers somehow 'let the show go on' thankfully!

February 2010:

Having tried a round of Clomid, I had a scan and it was discovered that I unfortunately suffered a side effect from it where the womb lining becomes too thin for that cycle. Apparently, this is fairly common. The conclusion therefore, was that sadly Clomid would not be a magical solution for us after all. I have however, since known friends where this has successfully worked for them so I would definitely recommend investigating it for other couples.

The next step we were informed should now be a recommended three rounds of IUI (artificial insemination). As previously explained, this entails me injecting myself daily for approximately two weeks with the hormone drug Gonal F, being scanned regularly to check on the developing eggs' sizes within my ovaries (an internal scan) and then over to Paul to produce his sperm sample at the peak time for me to ovulate. The sample is then injected inside my uterus. I won't pretend that any of this is going to be pleasant, dignified or fun. But frankly, if someone said, "Drink a glass of mud and you'll fall pregnant," I'd drink ten right now. In other words, as with all couples struggling to fall pregnant, I'm game for anything that could work.

Monday, 29th March 2010:

We have now embarked on two IUI's at The Lister. It's been a very difficult time. One of the difficult things with this situation that we've found ourselves in, is that you have to remain positive, upbeat and sure in your mind that it will work.

When it goes wrong and you're faced with another negative pregnancy test, you almost let yourself go; you have no reason to 'hold on to hope' now or stay positive. Your mind flashes back to all of the effort that you've just put in to the cycle (for approximately six weeks from beginning to pregnancy test), from the injections and diet to the regular journeys to and from the clinic.

The effort is tough. I remember injecting myself for the first time with pure fear. My hand was shaking as I drew this foreign object towards my tummy; I think I said to Paul 'I can't do it!' After he'd given me his supportive coaching words of wisdom, he left the room. Poor thing. I knew it's because he was upset at seeing me having to do this for us.

So having now had our second IUI, I did a pregnancy test (it's meant to be 14 days after the transfer procedure, but we couldn't wait and so it is actually 13 days today). Sadly, it was a big fat 'negative'; or as they call it on the fertility forums, a BFN.

For some reason, even though it feels like we have now taken about 100 pregnancy tests all saying 'negative' since we started trying, this second IUI cycle seems to have affected us both very badly. It must be all the added effort of the injections for a second time and the rollercoaster of hoping for nearly two weeks again that it had worked only to find it hadn't. Every breath you take and with every movement, your mind tells you what you're potentially 'carrying' and so it takes over your life night and day. You feel as though you need to have your tummy encased in bubble wrap!

As someone who is an optimist, I hate the fact that I can't stop feeling tearful today too (and I can see that my darling husband Paul is the same). And to top it all off, it feels as though everyone is currently having babies around us (from our cleaner to the Prime Minister to drug addicts on the news tonight)! How can this be?

Well, as usual, our way of coping is to put an action plan in place. Firstly, we are going to call our nurse at Dr Michael Dooley's office tomorrow to arrange our 3rd IUI at The Lister.

Fingers crossed (but not legs of course), we will be 3rd time lucky!

Monday, 5th April 2010 (Easter Monday):

So we're now on to our 3rd IUI cycle…it's pretty depressing stuff, but like I keep reminding myself, at least the doctors can offer us such a procedure these days.

Today is my 4th day of the Gonal F injections for this cycle.

It's amazing to think that I am almost becoming used to that 6 o'clock prick in my tummy! They tell you to gradually do it in the form of a smile around your belly button each night; one prick per night, and eventually they'll add up to a smile. This is to make sure you don't inject in to bruises…ironic, as believe me, there really is nothing to 'smile' about with this fertility game.

Never underestimate the emotion at every stage. The injections are tough…and I think I am becoming almost resentful that I am having to do them each night (as well as the fertility diet, the resting, which is hard while working full time editing and running the magazine and balancing family life, and of course now coping with side effects such as headaches, fatigue and feeling nauseous).

As good as your partner is trying to be towards you at this time too, I don't think at this stage they can fully understand how hard it is for the woman (who is not only going through this emotionally, but also physically). Your tummy feels constantly bloated and you have painful bruises across it. Plus, if you have a muscular tummy, it is even harder to find any fat to pinch thus avoiding the muscle (I'm afraid, being fairly slim, I have that problem). This is in no way a grumble at Paul, for he is being amazing; as is the small circle around me, who knows and cares about what we are going through. We decided to only tell our close family at this stage, namely our parents.

Last night at our Brighton Marina cocktail bar, there was a big party that the venue was playing host to. At the last hour, just before we were to get ready to go, I felt that I just couldn't party the night away. I had a bath, injected myself, and thought, *what on earth are you doing girl now going to a party?* After a small disagreement with Paul about it, he went alone. I really needed an early night and as my mother always says, "Sometimes you just need to listen to your body." We have to attend many events and launch parties. This was the first time I had ever missed one feeling like this. I know in time Paul will understand why I couldn't go.

I am disclosing this because couples need to expect that disagreements will happen when you're going through infertility, so don't be surprised; it is a traumatic time as a couple. It does not mean you're falling apart. It is just inevitable that you'll both cope in different ways and by doing different things to take you away from this terrible experience. You're both in the same boat, but you may wish to sail in different directions occasionally. And that's fine.

Anyway, I found Paul in the early hours staggering about in our bathroom. Yes, we all have our different ways of coping.

Tuesday, 6th April 2010:

We've just been to visit the nurse at Mr Dooley's office in The King Edward VII's Hospital London, for our initial scan for this new IUI cycle (though we are having the actual treatment in The Lister Hospital). We think that the reason they are doing this initial scan there is so that we get a more hands-on approach from

Mr Dooley's team (they could probably read the disappointment on our faces after the last cycle when we met with them afterwards).

Anyway, the news is that everything is looking good for this stage. And as is proving a pattern with me, there is one dominant follicle at the moment (however, everyone keeps telling me that one is all you need to get pregnant of course)! The size is 17 millimetres (there is another one that is 12 millimetres). The egg within a follicle is usually ripe when a follicle measures between 16 and 20 millimetres. Therefore, it looks as though I'll be having the procedure on Friday.

One thing that I am starting to struggle with now is that I'm so tired of being prodded around. And I keep worrying that Paul might think I'm too old, at 35; the age discussion with the nurse arose again! Unfortunately, with infertility, the woman's age is continuously discussed. So yes, it does bring you down. However, as one doctor reminded me recently, there is more and more evidence to show that the man's age also plays a significant role. So maybe one day such meetings will also discuss the man's age, then at least women won't feel like the age finger is only pointing at them if nothing else!

FACT BOX:

Follicles: An ovarian follicle is a roughly spheroid cellular set found in the ovaries.

It secretes hormones that influence stages of the menstrual cycle. Women begin

puberty with approximately 400,000 follicles, each with the potential to release

an egg cell (ovum) at ovulation for fertilization.

Wednesday, 7th April 2010:

I'm sitting on the train again going back up to London (that'll be two days running). The nurse from The Lister called me this morning to say that they would like to scan me again today and also instructed me to inject a higher dose of Gonal F last night (upon each visit and scan, you have a blood test for hormone levels which tells the doctor's whether you need more or less of the drugs. The results are received on the same day as the test is taken usually).

It is a chore travelling up to London all the time at the drop of a hat (and hard keeping it from everyone around me at work), but I'm in good hands at this hospital and they are at least monitoring me closely. I'm going alone this time as Paul couldn't make it due to prior work commitments, which is fine. There's no need for us to both keep popping up like this. Our businesses can't wait. We have some business stresses at the moment, and with this recession rearing its ugly head it doesn't help.

I might have a soak in a hot bath tonight to relax as once I've had the transfer, it is not advisable to have a hot bath for two weeks (only warm showers).

> **FACT BOX:** Hot baths, steam rooms, Jacuzzi's or showers can heat the body
>
> from the inside causing a high temperature, which is thought by some to cause
>
> miscarriage so is not usually recommended by most doctors.
>
> Some also recommend to avoid baths altogether and swimming, implying that
>
> showers are the safest option.
>
> Therefore, it is recommended to only have warm showers.

Friday, 9th April 2010:

Well, here it is, the day of our 3rd IUI transfer, procedure…and as ever, I'm nervous and apprehensive. I've discovered that you don't get used to it.

I'm on the train with Paul. It is a beautiful sunny day, so hopefully it will help to bring good things our way – fingers crossed.

Friday, 9th April 2010 (Post Transfer):

En route home now from having the IUI transfer at The Lister. Well, surprisingly, after dreading this one more than ever and feeling stupidly emotional about it today, it actually went really well. We had a kind nurse who we also met on our first visit to The Lister and remembered us (I think familiarity always makes a difference in these situations). I didn't feel a thing. She was very gentle and calming. Maybe this will be our '3rd time lucky' after all!

It's been the hottest day this year so far, so pre the transfer today, we had lunch in Hyde Park watching the ducks in the pond. I pray that our future child is reading this one day and can learn what a beautiful day it was.

It's so strange how when you have had the transfer, you become very aware that you're suddenly carrying this very precious little embryo or embryos inside of you that could potentially become you're much wanted baby. For me, every bump in the black cab on the way home and on the train becomes exaggerated in my mind. Due to heat being a possible factor for preventing pregnancy, you also become in tune with your body temperature and worry about that. Then you go through the paranoia of 'what if it falls out'? The reality is, if it's going to become a viable pregnancy, it will. But it's hard to convince yourself of this, as all you think to yourself is 'if there is anything I can do to help this embryo to hang in there, I will'!

So now, its home to carry on this 'baby making processes hopefully! We are now in the hands of the gods.

1st May 2010:

Well...very sadly, our 3rd IUI failed. My period decided to intervene by paying a visit a week early while we were on holiday in Egypt (we were advised by the doctors that it was fine to go away and that the relaxation may even help).

For some reason, this failure has hit us both very hard indeed! I feel like I spent much of the day on our hotel bed crying whenever I could vanish there alone. Poor Paul and Niomi; although I did put a brave face on to them, I am sure they could tell I was upset. Challenging times. And I feel so sorry for Paul too who I can tell it is affecting a lot now.

Mind you, I must say that despite that, we did manage to have a wonderful holiday altogether which really helped, in fact, one of our best family holidays (despite getting stuck for an extra week out there due to a volcanic ash cloud from Iceland that stopped a lot of flights including ours). It was the first time I did a deadline for the magazine remotely too! I think all of this commotion going on actually helped to take my mind off of the horrible failed cycle in the end. But never underestimate how tough this is.

I must now pick myself up again though, and find some inner strength to carry on.

So, now back in the UK, I am sat on the train again with Paul on our way up to London to discuss and start our 4th IUI at The Lister.

If this one fails, it's on to IVF (which as I've said before, terrifies me. I've never wanted to go down that route).

For this IUI, I have been given three different instructions for the Gonal F injections which was confusing, so I ended up choosing the dose myself.

5th May 2010:

Today, I had our 4th IUI transfer.

And what a horrible experience that one was. Three young nurses and the male doctor couldn't 'find my cervix'. Apparently, it may be because it was my first IUI procedure to take place in the morning and with the bladder not being so full, it doesn't press the cervix down in to place sometimes. There is so much to this biological stuff!

It was not a nice experience I must say! And I sensed that they were clearly a bit panicked themselves. It just wasn't happening. Paul was my rock as ever, holding my hand, keeping me calm (and rubbing my knees while they were nervously knocking against one other)!

15th May 2010:

As I took the pregnancy test on the Saturday just gone, I thought to myself, *if it says positive, I shall simply kiss that little testing stick*! Sadly (good for hygiene purposes though I suppose), it was another big fat nasty negative (or a BFN).

This is getting hard now. And, I'm aware that the path we've been led on to is only going to get harder. As well as all the emotions between us and our personal anger, Paul and I also have that feeling of 'why us', followed by guilt, because 'why not us'? We are so blessed in so many other ways (especially with Niomi). So we try to remind ourselves of that. People are going through far worse things in life, and that's what I keep telling myself at these dark moments of despair.

However, nothing takes away the fact or feeling that our hearts are praying for a baby together. I feel utter sadness too that I cannot give that to Paul. And so, each of the negative tests breaks our hearts a little bit more each month.

Today has also been a real palaver; one that we could have done without.

I rang our consultant, Michael Dooley, to inform him of the negative pregnancy test result from last week and to ask his advice on how we should now progress with IVF, but somehow I was passed around to several nurses, then to The Lister Hospital and then finally to Michael Dooley himself.

To cut a laboriously long story short, Paul and I had to drive everything forward ourselves. We ended up on Wimpole Street in London just a few hours later quickly having all the necessary blood tests that legally you have to have in place prior to IVF (from HIV to Hepatitis B to mention a couple. Another few hundred pounds thrown at this fertility game).

What a day!

We had made our minds up that we now had to go for the dreaded IVF and that now was the time. After all, time is of the essence with neither of us getting any younger.

Therefore, everything was suddenly a rush against time due to my cycle. It's all about the timing. You literally have to drop everything with this infertility saga.

So, the IVF route it is for us now. I could now write, "Yes, it'll be tough, but I'll be OK and it's worth it etc." But no, I have a confession…I am terrified. No, petrified. And of course, no, I don't know if it'll be worth it.

There, I've admitted it. I am a complete chicken. But will I let anyone know? Of course not! The smiles and 'the face' will be on as always. And it helps. I need to just get on and deal with it now.

I think that what scares me the most is the thought that I am (well, my body is) going in to the unknown now. And I always like to 'know'.

How will I react emotionally and physically to IVF? How long will the treatment be? Mentally will we both cope as a couple? And what if after all of that, we have another negative? I can't even contemplate that right now though. I must focus on positives.

I still receive comments that I need to 'just relax and then it'll happen'. While I, of course, know that they mean well, if anyone knows how to relax while facing this mental torture, while having needles prodded in them daily and suffering the side effects, please teach me (this is what I want to say anyway when I smile back politely). I know everyone means well, and I do appreciate that the few close family members that know what we are going through must struggle with what to say. I completely sympathise with that.

Well, I'm off now…to meet our new friend IVF. I'll let you know how we get on!

1st IVF Cycle
20th May 2010:

We were hoping we would be booked at The Lister Hospital.

I can honestly say that yesterday was one of the most
stressful days we've had so far on this journey. We were booked
for a scan at a London women's clinic, on Harley Street with an
appointment with Mr Dooley afterwards at his office. As the
timing with my cycle caused it to be a bit last minute, The Lister
were sadly fully booked. Meanwhile, due to a personal
emergency that he could not help, our appointment with Mr
Dooley was cancelled while we were in London.

To cut a long story short, we had to wait four hours at the women's clinic to get our prescriptions etc. With me being on day three of my cycle, if we couldn't get the medication, we would have missed this IVF cycle (and again, so much effort has gone in to the preparation). And then, with Paul going away to see the World Cup football next month in South Africa, we would have missed two months. We are both very aware that the clock is ticking.

So, after everyone running around all afternoon getting my first file underway, with our blood test results, we were finally given our protocol for IVF this month. The good news is that I don't need to do the down regulating (where the woman's body is basically shut down hormonally with drugs before it's rebooted. It basically depletes the pituitary gland from its hormones that controls ovulation. This can in turn cause menopausal symptoms). So I was pleased to avoid that part.

I now have to inject twice daily with Gonal F (same drug as for the IUI) and one other, Cetrotide, towards the end of the cycle.

I'm now on my way to meet Paul and the doctor at the London women's clinic. They seem very good and professional. I just wish it was as near as The Lister Hospital is for us to get to by taxi from Victoria Station. We didn't even know that we were not having our first IVF at The Lister until the end of yesterday's meeting with the London women's clinic.

The doctor explained to us that they have a 'special offer' on currently. Three IVFs for the price of two. I know, I can't believe it exists but it does; a bit crude we thought, like shopping in a supermarket! The costs are getting extreme now, with everything so far amounting to in excess of £10,000.

The clinic said we would probably need more than one cycle and that we are an obvious couple to opt for this 'special offer'. Since they are pushing us for this, I think we are now signing up for 'the special three for two'. How depressing. We are taking the risk of losing money, despite wishing that I will get pregnant on the first attempt. But we figured it is worth it as we could potentially save money on one free cycle, if needed. Believe me, the trouble with infertility is that you'll do anything. As intelligent people, you know this too but you still do it. Isn't that strange.

We have now spent months solidly on the internet looking up everything there is to know about infertility daily, driving ourselves mad with any glimmers of helpful advice. We constantly show each other things we've discovered, toying with 'hope'. From an 'Avocado diet reportedly being able to triple chances of success for couples undergoing IVF' in a newspaper article, to a Science Daily article on a 'new method for picking the right egg in IVF', we read and study everything we find! Staying positive through all of this is our safety net.

22nd May 2010:

I'm on my way up to the women's clinic with my mother and my daughter, Niomi (who we are dropping at Topshop on the way). My mother kindly volunteered to come with me.

What is also hard with IVF and fertility treatments is the time it takes up in your personal life. Fortunately, I work for myself, but it is stressful editing the magazine and doing deadlines while going through this. But I do sympathise so much for the women who have to book their 'holiday' time off to do such treatments. That must be terrible.

I'm getting used to this routine of catching the Gatwick Express, followed by a cab each day, then back again and then catching up on my work upon my return with my team (who of course don't know what I am going through).

This treatment can also mess with your mind so much and makes you question everything about yourself.

For example, at the meeting with our doctor at the London women's clinic two days ago with Paul, I went in to it feeling about 20 years old (largely due to the kind nurse telling me beforehand that I am still so young so I mustn't worry) and came out feeling about 100! He kept informing us that my AMH level was low. As if I needed reminding. It's 8.5 currently. Yes it's low-ish (ideal is approx. 12), but it's not *that* bad. And it's slightly higher than it once was!

Anyway, one good thing was that on this first scan I've just had for this cycle, I have 8 follicles on each side; more than they had anticipated for me (and 8 is our lucky number – we were married on 8/8/8).

41

30th May 2010:

Well, it's only been a few days since I last wrote in here but so much has happened, and I have not felt strong enough to pen it down.

After a second scan with the same doctor, we saw previously at the London women's clinic (who was very nice and even said this time that he thought I'm still young – he must have felt bad after last time) it was decided that I had only 3 dominant follicles and so I was booked to have them retrieved last Saturday.

Niomi's 18th birthday was on the Wednesday which, needless to say, was so important to me so we carried on with her birthday plans as normal, going to London the night before the procedure on the Friday for dinner at London haunt, Sketch, and then even for a quick dance at Mahiki as she'd so wanted to go there (it's the hip place to go in London at the moment). It was actually all great for me as it completely took my mind (and Paul's) off what would be happening the following morning and so it calmed my nerves. And most importantly, Niomi had a fabulous time! Needless to say, no alcohol was consumed by us and we managed to be in our hotel bed by midnight! I wondered if I'm the only woman to have been there the night before such a procedure. It made me chuckle to myself. My advice at this stage though, is to carry on with life as normally as you possibly can. If you feel like doing things, do them. If you don't, then give in and do nothing.

Going out and having some fun was also nice for Niomi so that she could relax and enjoy her birthday as she has been working so hard lately; she's at college taking her A and AS Levels. She's a hard worker. I've always had to literally drag her away from her study books to encourage her to take a break!

Unfortunately, the op didn't go well…at all. Well, the op itself did, but I was taken ill immediately afterwards – very ill. It began with me fainting when I got back to my bed and then I was vomiting continuously and uncontrollably. The nurse called for help and turned my bed nearly vertical with my head down so I was almost upside down; this was because my blood pressure had also dropped dangerously low. The room that I had been put in after the procedure was a shared area unfortunately, very old-fashioned with just a curtain dividing me from other patients.

This is all they have at this clinic – very primitive indeed. We could all hear each other's results which was not a good experience. And now, they could hear me being taken ill.

I was in full view of all the other patients and their partners departing the ward. They all looked at me as they passed by – I must have looked dreadful and pale. I felt very vulnerable. I remember hearing one patient (who I gather was a student donating her eggs for some extra cash) informing the nurse when she came round, "I feel great! I'll definitely be recommending this to all of my friends at uni!" It was a bizarre scenario that I didn't know happened. Meanwhile, a couple who were both in beds close to mine (yes, men often need procedures as well) were visited by my nurse. She then returned and very loudly announced to Paul and I, "He is a very fat man next door to you, so it's taken me ages to find a vein in his arm!" We were so shocked and embarrassed for him; on top of the humiliation of what this poor man was going through, he would have heard what she had said to us. It wasn't professional or kind.

We also then heard the same nurse complaining on the phone to a colleague, (or maybe a friend) "I've had one taken really ill today so now I've got to work late till she's better." It was me she was talking about. She sounded quite irritated. Was there no compassion in this place?

My mother was with us by then as she'd joined us in London the previous night. I just kept saying that I wanted to get out of this place now and be at home.

Somehow, Paul and my mother managed to get me dressed and in to my stepfather Ian's car who was waiting outside once my blood pressure had returned to normal and my sickness had stopped. However, when we were in the car a mile or two away from the clinic, I fainted and then couldn't stop vomiting again, and felt hot and in a daze. Suddenly, I didn't know where I was. My family quickly drove me back to the clinic where I had to continue recovering for another few hours.

We weren't given an explanation why this happened to me; was it a reaction to the anaesthetic or was I given too high a dose of something?

I recall it had been a very strange set up in the operating room. I remember a nurse telling off another nurse because she had not tied my long hair back. There was definite tension in the room which didn't really help me relax. It was as if I wasn't there! Paul also commented that when he had to go off to 'do his business' (collect his sperm), he had to walk through a room full of young receptionists with his sample in his hand – again not very professional. And not very nice for the men doing this; there was no privacy.

That was all yesterday, and I've since started to recover slowly today. I've also now learnt that my blood pressure had dropped down to 66/38, and apparently the '38' was what was concerning them.

Anyway, first thing this morning we had a call from the embryologist to say that out of the three eggs taken two are doing very well. We also opted for ICSI at this stage (which means Paul's sperm is injected directly in to the egg apparently giving us a better chance, as opposed to standard IVF where basically the sperm is left to 'find an egg' in a dish).

So to summarise, today I was back in the clinic for the embryo transfer. I was still feeling very shaky and not 100% at all, so it wasn't exactly easy. I was on autopilot. But nevertheless, it's now done. And the doctors and nurses seem to think that we have a very good chance now as in the UK they only ever put two fertilised embryos back anyway. Therefore, we are now on the same plane as everyone else.

Now we have the 2 week wait followed by the nerve-wracking pregnancy test.

It has been a traumatic couple of days. And I'm shattered. It's now time to rest, and as advised after all transfers, I must now drink two litres of water per day.

June 12ᵗʰ 2010 (also my birthday):

Well, the crazy rollercoaster continues. After much deliberating, Paul and I felt that we'd take the gamble and do the pregnancy test today as it's 2 weeks to the day since egg retrieval. Also, it being my birthday today, we thought it may bring us some luck. Not a good idea. It was a BFN. Feel a bit shell-shocked and of course very, very sad for us both. What can we say to each other, other than that we love each other and cuddle lots (which is what we do every time…and cry)?

It seems so unfair, even more so after I suffered so badly after the operation for this attempt. I convinced myself that something good would come of it and that being my birthday, this would be our happy ending.

I've also been so extra good on my healthy eating. I've drunk my two litres of water per day, drunk lots of green tea (which is meant to help improve egg quality), and have eaten copious amounts of almonds, raspberries, avocado and plenty of pineapple (which is meant to assist in implantation).

On top of that, I've tried to be positive...even when I've received such comments as I have recently from people asking if I'm pregnant yet? It all hurts so much. And even a close friend who is aware of what we are going through lightly patted my (empty) tummy last week and cheerfully asked, "Any baby news for me yet? Hurry up, baby." I know they meant well. It just hurts so much and I find myself stumbling on my words as I answer, but I've been strong and still tell myself 'it will happen', until now. I now find myself wondering if it will after all?

Well, I know this self-pity is selfish and does no good, but I need to sometimes let off steam privately to myself.

I know it may be wrong too, but since taking the pregnancy test today, I'm also holding out a 5% hope since my period hasn't arrived yet. Today is Saturday, so if it still does not appear by Monday, Paul and I have agreed that we will test again then.

2nd IVF Cycle
29th July 2010:

There's so much to catch up on since my last entry. Sadly, my period did arrive after all and so it was a definite negative result after my first IVF cycle.

Nearly 2 weeks ago, I had our 2nd attempt at IVF. Yes, just as with the previous one, we had the same fears and emotions, but also this time I was put to sleep with a general anaesthetic due to the reactions I previously suffered. Well, to cut a long story short, the whole procedure went a lot better in that I'm still here feeling fine (a bonus) and didn't take a funny turn. It's very hard for Paul though I'm sure witnessing me being taken off to theatre, especially after what happened last time.

The bad part though, is that I only had one embryo that was viable to be put back. This is really concerning us. It's also incredibly frustrating and disheartening. An emotion you just can't understand unless you've experienced the effort of IVF.

I do the pregnancy test on 31st July (ironically, it's Paul's birthday this time)!

However, we are at the airport today on our way to Spain (just as with the IUI, the doctor said flying makes no difference) for Paul's surprise birthday holiday…and I hate to admit this, but I think my period may have just started. I just feel it. I am so worried. And I don't want to tell Paul as it'll spoil our journey. I'm so worried.

I feel so sad, but I am putting on a brave face. I keep finding myself asking time and time again, "Why us?" We love each other so very much, I think we are good people, we are both eating all that we should…so, why?

5th August 2010:

Sadly, two days after writing in here, my period did arrive. Even though I convinced myself it was coming, it's still always a terrible shock; something you cannot control and you hate it when it happens.

Even though we've now had so many setbacks, it's still very hard and each negative is tougher and harder to accept as time goes by.

I felt it was especially hard for Paul this month initially. He was desperately sad, which I absolutely hate seeing, and I cannot do anything about it. And me? Well, for some reason this time I felt numb and almost blasé as if to say 'again…I'm not surprised'. I was fed up!

However, as the days have gone by, it's now become harder than ever before for me. I have felt like I'm in a very dark place, wondering if I'll ever become pregnant. This isn't like me, so I hate these negative feelings. What usually keeps us going is that we are both optimists in life.

Tears keep coming to my eyes and streaming down my face…even as I write this (and we are on our flight home now). This is my lowest ebb.

Considering what's happened, we somehow managed to have a really nice holiday in between this rubbish; once again, it helps to put a 'face on'. I think that being away, helped us in many ways as it preoccupied us most of the time.

I feel guilty too though; guilt has really set in inside me. I feel as though it is my fault that we can't or won't be able to have children together, despite the professionals telling us that we are in the 'unexplained category' which really means there is no known reason for our infertility. That in itself is hard though. Since if we knew what was wrong, we may be able to have treatment and correct it.

Yesterday, we met with friends on our holiday; three couples we know with 10 children between them and a new baby. All we want is one together. It is so hard at times. And I feel selfish saying that. Mind you, being with other people's children or babies is not hard for us in the sense that as we always say 'they are not ours'. For us, it is more the seeing a family set-up that is difficult just because it reminds us of what we are missing. I adore, and always have, children and babies of all ages. I always thought I'd have five children. How foolish was I?

So, it's back to normal life for us for now. Personally, I find it helps to just plunge myself back in to my work and find a focus away from this when it's this hard (although I do then find myself trawling the internet for some 'miracle' potion or procedure out there). The usual staff issues brought to your attention can also seem so mundane, especially for example if you have a member of staff off sick with a simple cold. But if nothing else, such irritancies take my mind off of everything in the infertility world!

For me, I find that it really helps to work out at the gym too. I go twice per week to my personal trainer. It's a very important time for me to escape and so it's a salvation in many ways. Having said that, whenever I am at the end of an IVF cycle, I have a break for a while as by then my tummy is bloated and then once a transfer has been done, as I mentioned previously, it is not advisable to allow the body to get to a high temperature. And I am sure exercising would not help at that stage anyway. Fortunately, my personal trainer is very understanding as he had his daughter through IVF and is very open and knowledgeable about it. It is amazing how when (and if) you do open up a little bit about infertility, so many people have either been through it themselves or are going through it.

Life and making new life is the biggest thing in the world, and yet we struggle as a society to discuss it. Strange that, isn't it?

3rd IVF Cycle
25th August 2010:

I'm on my way up to London on the train…again. Today will be my first scan of our 3rd IVF cycle (from the special offer at the London women's clinic).

Yes, treatment commences once again and this month (well, running up to this cycle) I have literally tried everything, read up on everything and Googled everything looking for that miracle that could increase our chances. I'm now taking Royal Jelly capsules daily, as well as continuing to drink copious amounts of green tea and eating almonds all day long (and I am still taking folic acid daily)!

Last week, we had another meeting with Dr Michael Dooley who assured us that contrary to what we were recently told by another doctor (at the London women's clinic), we should keep going. We are, after all, in the 'unexplained' category (frustrating to say the least, but I guess it gives us hope).

Since writing the previous entry, we both hit rock bottom with a bang.

We had a follow up meeting with the doctor who performed the last IVF at the London women's clinic. The news from her was bad and unexpected; we were not prepared for what she said. She informed us that since the egg results (how many were being produced) and the quality of the eggs were 'not good' in the last cycle, our chances of conceiving, even through IVF, were now 5% and that we should consider egg donors (something I respect works for a lot of women/couples, but a route I really do not ever want to go down, and simply cannot). She said that my eggs were 'black' and that basically meant they would never fertilise. She told us it was not worth us having this final 'free' IVF cycle with her clinic. She did, however, say that if we decide to try using donor eggs with them, we would have to pay for that IVF cycle (as well as the donor eggs of course – in other words, it would be a more expensive route).

We sat in the meeting with her while she spoke very matter-of-factly about our future; we were in tears. She then left us alone to sob in her office until we could compose ourselves to leave.

We were shell-shocked. Stupidly perhaps, we never considered this would be the end. Or that it would end like this; by a doctor just coming out with it. But it appeared this was 'the end'.

A nurse then came and took us to a 'quiet room' next door prepared with boxes of tissues. Obviously, this room was for people being given such news. We just sat and wept and wept. Our bodies shook with our sobs. Every time one of us composed ourselves to leave, the other one sobbed harder again.

After a while, we departed the building on Harley Street in a daze without anyone saying good-bye to us. As we stepped outside, the world seemed like a different place.

We walked to the end of Harley Street to a nearby park and held hands still crying and crying. We were now in pieces. And yet, the rest of the world was carrying on as normal around us which was a strange feeling.

In the park, Paul did touch on the delicate subject of asking me if I would consider egg donors with his sperm. I explained with sorrow that it was something I just felt I couldn't do. We are all different and I fully respect other people's opinions on this subject, but it isn't something I can do. It's a personal choice. Even IVF is further than I thought I could go. I now knew deep down I had to accept, it was all over. In addition, once I explained to Paul that an egg donor baby would not have my DNA, he sobbed even more and declared that he only ever wanted *my* baby. Perhaps it was the shock of the news we had just been given, but he had not realised I would just be carrying the baby; it would not biologically be mine.

Now, as well as the pain I felt, I also felt guilt that my 'black' eggs had prevented Paul from having children. But how come I had my daughter?

Something started to tell me this was wrong.

After a few days of being back at work and carrying on as normal, the shock started to settle slightly (the pain was still raw though). And as it began to settle, we started to ask ourselves why the embryologist who worked on our first IVF told us that the eggs were 'excellent quality'? Could my body have really changed that much within a few short months? And therefore, considering the apparent quality of the eggs from that first cycle, should we really just give up?

So, we went to see Dr Michael Dooley again. As I mentioned above, he insisted that we still had a good chance and that if we were happy to continue, we should keep trying. I think he could see how desperate we were to have a child together. Needless to say, I am sure he is sadly used to informing couples of the tragic news that it will never happen. So with this in mind, we were feeling a bit more positive again at what he was telling us.

In the meantime, he has written to the embryologist at the London women's clinic asking for full reports on both of our two previous IVF cycles.

So this rollercoaster has continued, with a few scary dives on it.

Today is now the first scan of this 3rd IVF cycle and tonight I begin the injections again (the same higher dose as the previous cycle).

Fingers are crossed as always…and we are praying.

10th September 2010:

Once again, so much has happened since my last entry.

The embryologist kindly called me during my treatment of this, our 3rd cycle, and informed me that the egg quality on the first IVF was actually just 'OK' and that on the second the quality was 'poor'.

She was very sympathetic to how hard this news was for me, and when she realised I was currently being treated she said that I must now forget all of that and stay calm focusing on this new cycle.

Paul and I figured for ourselves out how much of the drug Gonal F I should inject for this cycle, since we realised it was possible that the high dose over a short period of time that I was given in the previous cycles could actually be damaging my egg quality each time; a high dose was possibly 'cooking' me too quick thus damaging my egg quality. We discovered that this can happen simply through my gut instinct (followed by Googling it to see if there was any evidence for this). Sure enough, there was. For some women, this short burst approach can damage the egg quality; this could be what the so-called 'black egg' damage was.

There was enough evidence for us to request that the London women's clinic put me on 225 IU per day as opposed to the 450 IU they had put me on previously. Dr Michael Dooley also agreed with us that this was worth a try. Why hadn't the London women's clinic figured this out though? We are meant to be the novices.

One good thing a nurse from the clinic informed us, was that the expensive drugs required for IVF cycles are a lot cheaper at ASDA supermarket of all places. So rather than going to a chemist or a pharmacy within a clinic, we bought ours this month from the local ASDA at Brighton Marina (in their pharmacy I might add, not in the fruit and veg section)!

You would think that as time goes by the injections in to your tummy would become easier…they don't. In fact, if anything, they have become harder for me. Perhaps it's what they represent emotionally, every single one a reminder of what we are going through. With each one, I say a prayer and hope beyond hope.

During my first scan of this cycle, we were fortunate to have the most wonderful and caring nurse called Louise who was new at the clinic. She had thoroughly read all of my notes prior to us arriving. This was a first for us at this clinic as we usually had to give our full story again and again to each nurse at every scan, which was tiresome. She informed us how she had only ever seen a case like ours once before and the lady produced better quality eggs on the lower dose! We were now feeling this had been the right decision. However, she hadn't yet performed our scan. We braced ourselves as the invasive scan began.

It appeared our theory was working! We had seven follicles…yes seven (as oppose to our usual 1s, 2s or 3s).

Louise was so caring throughout, taking time to ask how we both were.

Since then, I've had subsequent scans for this cycle every other day, continued treatment for a massive great 11 days (usually I'm 'cooked' after five days) and then two days ago I had my egg collection operation.

We had a wonderful eight eggs retrieved! Our magic number 8.

We were overjoyed…even though the experience was quite a comic fiasco. I was moved from one bed to another twice for some reason, and then when I was being given my drip for the general anaesthetic and I mentioned that I had a splinter in the back of my hand, the nurse nearly screamed at me and said, "You should have informed us before. You could have died if it got infected. I will ask the doctor if you can still have this done!" Panic set in as we waited. She then returned, appearing quite stern, and said, "OK, you can have it." I fear she overreacted. To ask for any sympathy to calm my shaking nerves would have been far too much I could tell. I just went along with her Sergeant Major-style instructions and got on with it.

Anyway, the results were not bad for the couple told a few weeks ago that I would only ever produce poor egg numbers and quality, and that we should use, or should I say 'purchase', donor eggs!

Meanwhile, having received great A Level grades from college, Niomi is off to university to study law in a couple of weeks. It's an exciting (and nerve-wracking) time of change, and we have lots to prepare. Last week I took her shopping in London to get all the bits she will need in her campus. I'll miss her so much!

11th September 2010 (Day after Egg Collection):

My stomach has felt bloated and uncomfortable and painful this time after egg collection. The pain also seems to be worse today than yesterday strangely. It's especially bad on my right hand side, deep down and swollen.

Fortunately, we are currently on our way to the clinic now to have the embryo transfer so I will inform them of how I am feeling this time and ask if it is normal (especially as I have a strong pain threshold).

As ever, Paul is my rock!

20th September 2010:

Today, Paul and I dropped Niomi to university in Bristol for the first time. It was extremely emotional; even more than I expected.

It's a strange feeling, because while you feel so immensely proud, you're also very aware that this is the beginning of your child really growing up and the first step to leaving home (well, almost. I'll make sure she always has a bedroom at home)!

Paul and I acted 'cool' the whole time, trying to keep Niomi relaxed as this was such a huge episode in her life that she was embarking upon. We understood fully that although she was acting fine (I wonder where she gets that from!) she must have been very nervous. So, Paul and I promised ourselves before we left the house that we wouldn't cry.

Well, unfortunately that went completely out of the window when after spending the day setting up her room etc., we departed with her to the communal lift to take us downstairs. Paul and I hugged her in there, and then tears that I had been holding in all day came streaming down my face (which then triggered Paul also). Niomi kept saying, "Wipe your faces, someone may see you." Then the lift stopped suddenly at a floor to let in a bunch of teenage girls. They politely introduced themselves to Niomi…and Niomi (knowing we now looked a state) reluctantly said, "These are my parents." We smiled and smudged our tears away! I hope she'll forgive us one day and just put it down to another embarrassing parent moment!

26th September 2010:

After our most hopeful procedure yet, and then the worst and most intense two week wait so far, my dreaded period unexpectedly arrived in abundance three days ago.

To say that this hit us both hard, is a massive understatement.

With the results appearing so perfect this time (the embryo quality, the amount retrieved, my lining being thicker than usual) we had probably convinced ourselves that this was our time and that it had worked.

So much so that even when I started to bleed, we still hoped that it was just what is called 'embedding bleed'. We were in complete denial.

So what now? Financially, as well as emotionally, this journey has become a fraught experience. Most of the time now I feel like I am on another planet and that this is just a horrible nightmare.

28ᵗʰ September 2010:

Dr Michael Dooley called me to see how we were today. He is amazing the way that he keeps in touch with us by calling or texting or emailing; and he is a busy man being one of the top consultants in the UK. We can tell that he is genuinely very sympathetic to us. He said it is also 'bad luck' since, if anything, our results are improving as time goes by.

He agrees that our decision to inject a lower dose of Gonal F over a longer period of time obviously agrees with me more. I guess in a sense it wasn't a completely wasted experience, as now we at least know that this protocol suits me.

So after much deliberating and sleepless nights thinking hard, we've told Michael (as he said he prefers us to call him) that we would like to continue in this world of IVF. The truth is, neither of us is ready to give up. Something keeps telling us that one day we will have a baby together.

Mind you, on a practical note, we must also be careful not to lose too much money over this. Each cycle costs in the region of £6000, plus there are our added travel costs (approx. £100 per visit) and blood tests (anything from £200 – thousands of pounds). And then, of course there are other day to day expenses such as Niomi's university and our businesses.

We informed Michael that we were not impressed with the set up or care at the London women's clinic and in retrospect thought it was a bit strange selling us a '3 for 2' supermarket-style package (especially as they then suggested we shouldn't use the final 'free' cycle).

So, Michael has booked us in to The Lister Hospital in Chelsea where we had our initial IUIs and were very happy there.

This will be our fourth IVF cycle; words I thought I'd never say.

In the meantime, Michael has also suggested that I have a few extra blood tests (in addition to the mountain of IVF bloods) that will check for such things as immunity issues, including NK

Cells (natural killer cells) which is when cells prevent an embryo developing as they think it is an anti-body which they attack. However, you live a normal life not being aware you have them, as there are often no symptoms. If they are found, steroids are prescribed during the IVF cycle to keep them at bay. The downside is that this simple blood test alone costs £800 done privately!

However, today I visited my GP and asked whether the NHS can help us at all with any such blood tests that we now require. We had of course already been informed by my GP that since I already have a child, we are not entitled to any help or IVFs from the NHS. However, Michael said it was worth asking if they would help with these blood tests. So, I went along with my list.

Thankfully, my GP said he was happy to carry out any tests that he could and he was extremely apologetic that he couldn't help any further; his hands are clearly tied by the system in our area. He was also extremely sympathetic at the amount we had run up in the fertility world (hitting approximately £20,000 now).

So tomorrow, I am hopefully having the blood tests and then when my next period starts the next IVF at The Lister begins.

FACT BOX:

NK cells stands for natural killer cells.

Natural killer cells in the blood are naturally occurring and play a vital part in the immune system. They are lymphocytes (white blood cells) which are produced in the bone marrow, spleen and other parts of the body before circulating in the blood. Their purpose is to recognize and target cells which do not belong to the body, e.g. tumors, viruses, bacteria. They are also important in the adaptive immune response, whereby the body becomes immune to infections it has previously encountered.

Natural Killer cells in the uterus appear to have similar features to those in the blood but their role is unknown; it is believed that they may play a part in mediating the maternal-fetus interface of the placenta. It is thought by some doctors and scientists today that NK cells play a large part in causing some miscarriages since it is possible they may detect a fetus as a foreign body or disease and therefore try to rid the body of it.

5ᵗʰ October 2010:

Coping with the heartache and emotional stress during your month off from IVF before commencing a new cycle, as I've discovered, is hard.

What I am learning, is that each failure hits you harder…you blame yourself and question everything that you did from what you ate and drank to what you even thought. I find myself asking torturous questions such as, "Maybe it was that morning cup of tea with caffeine in it? Did I have too much stress this month? Was it that magazine deadline I had?" The reality is, when you've had a perfect IVF cycle that doesn't work, no one has the answer; not even the professionals. And that makes it even more difficult to deal with. The unknown.

I'm also continuing to learn that we all cope in different ways. For example, I just want to go in to hiding for now, cuddled up watching TV in comfort whereas I think Paul would prefer to be out with people forgetting about it. No one way is the right way.

I'm even struggling seeing people in general, which isn't like me. I'm so used to going to launch parties, interviewing important people and having meetings. It sounds awful, but I am avoiding anyone except Paul, Niomi and my parents this week. Part of me thinks I will just wait until I have some 'good news'. Praying.

But as a result, you can by your own doing risk feeling quite alone on this journey. But then, IVF is a lonely world. It still has such a stigma attached to it. And so with the physical and emotional pain that you have to go through, you have no choice but to keep all of this to yourself. And somehow 'smile' whenever you do get the courage to see people. And I can be a good actress when needed!

Fortunately, I have in particular two great friends that I can confide in. They've both been my confidantes. One has also been through a similar experience, as well as simply being a supportive person to me. Recently at a friend's book launch, one of these dear friends simply turned to me and said, "Are you OK?" I nodded that I was actually fine. She quietly said, "If you need to pop outside, let me know and we'll escape together." You need your friends at times like this.

10ᵗʰ October 2010:

We are currently on a plane on our way to Spain with my mother and stepfather, Ian, for a week's break before embarking upon our 4ᵗʰ IVF.

This is the trip that we were supposed to take after our 3ʳᵈ IVF, but as it ended up being a longer protocol cycle than expected we had to alter our flights to now.

We are both really looking forward to getting away, and I'm looking forward to getting my body prepared and ready for the next lot of treatment. Some autumn sunshine and swimming is the perfect medicine I am sure! Fortunately, as it is my parent's property, it is like home from home for us too. We plan to relax as much as possible. Also, since my mother and stepfather know what we are going through, there is no pressure; we can just be ourselves.

Although, being at the airport today surrounded by families with babies made me realise that while we are away we will be seeing a lot of such reminders; and that's just what they are, reminders. You can be having a lovely time forgetting everything, and then 'bam' you see an adorable baby or doting parents and suddenly you're taken back to the pain. And this can happen anywhere. It sounds very selfish, but when you are going through IVF or simply infertility, every time you see a baby, a pregnant woman or families it simply reminds you of what you're going through and how you feel your body is 'broken'; or at least, that's how I feel at the moment. It's not that you long for anyone else's baby or child, or feel jealousy towards them, it's just the 'reminder' of this turmoil. Mind you, we are both so good at putting on an act; anyone who knows us will be quite surprised if they read this. But sometimes in awkward situations, such as being asked if we have children together yet, we glance knowingly at each other and Paul will squeeze my hand as we find an awkward way of saying 'no'. So frequently, we are also asked, "When are you going to have a baby?" I've even had people tell me, "You should hurry up and get on with it!" We just can't bring ourselves to embarrass them by explaining: "Actually, we wish we could, we are currently going through hell trying!" And then, there are the times when we just let people assume we don't want a baby together.

Last week in London, there was a lady struggling on the escalators at the tube station with a pram; no one was helping her. I nudged Paul who then promptly ran to assist her. We looked at each other and I said to him, "One good deed deserves another!" We always hope.

4th IVF Cycle

3rd November 2010 (Day of Egg Collection):

Dawn is breaking and Paul and I are sitting on a train to Victoria, London, again for our attempt number four at IVF. Today is the day of egg collection, and due to my health problems that occurred with the first cycle at the London women's clinic, The Lister Hospital have said that they would prefer me to be the first patient to go in today so that I can eat and drink soon after coming around from the general anaesthetic.

Having this cycle at The Lister has made a massive difference emotionally to us so far. It is a much more professional and caring environment.

I've also produced seven large follicles and four smaller ones (11 in total!), which is much better than in the past cycles. So much for the doctor at the London women's clinic who told us that I would 'never produce more that 1 or 2 eggs' and that we should give up and use donors (more expensive funnily enough)!

Well, here goes with cycle number four, my eighth fertility procedure if including the IUIs. I'll be going under my general anaesthetic in a couple of hours hopefully. Nervous, but being positive as always!

FACT BOX:

General anesthetic during IVF- For me, a general anesthetic worked extremely well. I never would have believed that, since you imagine it to be much harsher than a sedative (which is the other option at some hospitals). In fact, when I was put in to a semi-conscious state, I actually found that my body struggled to get back to its normal self again. Also, the procedure of egg collection is not a nice one to imagine, so it is of an advantage to be asleep.

8th November 2010:

Well, it was five days ago now and the procedure went well; in fact, very well indeed. I have also been feeling better recovering quicker than usual. I even attended a three-hour meeting at one of our businesses yesterday. Of course, as always, no one around us has a clue.

The floor that we were based on at The Lister was a world away from the rather barbaric Victorian-looking shared ward at The London Women's Clinic.

On arrival, we were taken up in a lift by a friendly porter to our private room, which was more like a hotel suite. It had a view across The Thames and a private en-suite bathroom, TV and even Molton Brown bottles everywhere. This was more like it.

We had privacy, it was clean and the staff were incredibly caring and professional; from the doctors to the nurses and even the anaesthetist.

We relaxed and watched morning TV and even ordered food from the menu for later. They placed me on a drip to hydrate me.

Then after the procedure, I wasn't too bad at all compared to previous experiences.

Paul was amazing as ever. It must be so hard for him watching me go through this. He's so strong and caring, and that helps me all the more. He keeps asking me if he can do anything for me. Several times, he's even asked if I can really keep going through this. Never underestimate how difficult this is for partners of the woman having fertility treatment.

I asked him to look after my phone as the porter took me off on the trolley and left him a message on the screen saying 'I'll be fine. Please don't worry. Love you x.'

So, the results? Well, the outcome was the best so far! They managed to retrieve 10 follicles. We were called that afternoon to be informed that nine were 'mature', which out of 10 is fantastic. The embryologist even visited us in our room after the procedure and explained the results in detail to us. She said she was very pleased so far. Another embryologist had also apparently spent about 20 minutes with Paul when I was in the operating theatre explaining various options open to us. What an informative and impressive place. These people actually cared about us as individuals.

The following day, we got the call from the embryologist; 10 were now all mature and all were A1 quality. Fantastic news! Of these, eight apparently looked like they were already fertilising well. Our magic number 8 again.

So we are booked in provisionally for a three-day transfer, but if things improve even more we may go to blastocyst (this is when the embryo's selection is viable to go to five or six days in the laboratory being monitored so that a selection of the best can be made. Two should become what are called blastocysts by then and can be put back. In the UK, no more than two can be put back. Basically, we would be overjoyed if we ever get to the blastocyst stage).

We were so happy with the results and this phone call.

And now? Well, I am so proud and ecstatic to say that we are on the train en route for a blastocyst transfer. Yes, we made it to the elite blastocyst club! We're absolutely thrilled and shocked. And nervous, as we know that we now have even higher hopes!

One thing on my mind though away from this, is that we do currently have some massive staff and business worries; this recession is hellish for our business sectors. And on top of that, the night before my egg collection, one of my photographers at our magazine decided to pull out of a fashion shoot I had planned for the next morning (he decided he didn't want to take direction on the style I had chosen). The shoot had 10 people involved who were travelling from all over England, some staying in hotels. Needless to say, this caused a lot of stress for me and needed a lot of phone calls that I really could have done without the night before my procedure! I managed to sort it out in the end though and the shoot went ahead as planned thank goodness. But that's what's difficult with infertility treatments; no one knows you're going through it (even if you had tooth ache you could say) and so the normal world around you carries on as usual, which can be more pressurised when running your own businesses; the magazine world is notoriously an especially stressful business to be in too.

23rd November 2010:

Well, to cut to the chase, sadly for some unknown reason the blastocysts did not take; we suffered another disappointing and gut-wrenching negative on a pregnancy test.

We can't quite believe it and can't understand what went wrong again. Having the embryos put back was as pleasant experience as is possible this time.

The doctor, nurse and embryologist were extremely kind and calming. They even played some classical music throughout the process which I personally think helps a person to relax (your legs are in stirrups and it is like having an invasive smear test, so anything that will help to relax you is a bonus).

Therefore, I felt that this time I was in a calm state, as was Paul; a world away from our previous clinic.

So after the transfer of the blastocysts, we departed for home convinced this was our time.

So now, I am on the train (meeting Paul in London as he's already there for a business meeting) so that we can meet with our doctor at The Lister Hospital to discuss what we do now, to see how we are and what could have gone wrong this time. A nurse has already explained over the phone to me that for unknown reasons embryos can simply decide to 'arrest' and give up.

Paul and I, as always, have a list of questions that include queries about various tests we've read about on the internet that we wonder if we should have.

We have also got to the stage where we have now spent in the region of £28k plus since starting this journey! Not good, especially during a recession. So this is an added worry; more cost that we really can't afford. But at the same time, this is our dream and we are only on this planet once. We can't bring ourselves to give up.

We think we will now have a break though, and decide what to do and when to regroup with our medical team.

5th IVF Cycle
7th May 2011:

This journey seems to be never ending. Having had a break from it all for a few months, we've decided to give the IVF world another push.

During this break, we have both felt that we are getting older, time is slipping by and it feels hopeless just doing nothing. Therefore, we decided to give it another go. We also felt that as we have tried so many times now, we must be getting closer to it actually working one day. Paul especially looks at the statistics and says the odds must be getting better with each attempt.

The Lister is the only place that we will consider having IVF from now on.

Meanwhile, Niomi is doing extremely well at university. We visit her regularly; she even cooked a meal for us on our last visit. Maybe that student cookbook that I sent to her has paid off! She seems to be a natural and is enjoying living there and fending for herself which is lovely to witness. It's so nice for me to see her thrive so well down there; she seems very happy which all I can ask for is. She's a very conscientious girl so I am sure she will do well too.

So here we are embarking on our 5th IVF cycle. The results so far are as follows:

1st May 2011: First scan=eight follicles. Four each side.
3rd May 2011: Second scan=five big and three smaller.
5th May 2011: Third scan=six big ones and two small.
7th May 2011 (today): Fourth scan=seven now ready and big. One is 13.5 mm so may grow by Monday when egg collection happens. Paul is always amazed at how large the follicles actually are inside a tummy at this stage. 'Like a group of large marbles' is how one nurse explained it to us. No wonder I feel bloated.

Talking of 'marbles', a funny thing happened today. While in London, I thought I'd pop along to Harrods to buy a friend a birthday present. Anyway, on my way I stopped to 'window shop' at a jeweller on Brompton Road (by Harrods). As I approached the window, on the packed street full of tourists and the like, a large chunky pearl necklace that I was wearing spontaneously snapped sending all of the marble-sized pearls flying across the pavement. The whole area stopped…everyone was suddenly scrambling about picking up and catching my pearls as they bounced up and down the pavement, passing handfuls of them to me. I kept politely telling everyone there really was no need, to stop, and informing them that they weren't actually real pearls either! But even after that rather embarrassing episode as I walked in to Harrods grinning at what had just occurred, a young Spanish boy came running up to me shouting, "Hola, hola, señora," and handed me a few more 'pearls' he had caught. It was quite a fiasco! But a lovely incident too, heart-warming, and in contrast to everything currently going on in my life!

Then I noticed the shop Zara was next to Harrods, which is where my necklace was incidentally from. I thought it's worth informing them what had just happened. Even with no receipt, the manager kindly changed it for me to a new one, she obviously took pity upon my story of the episode outside that I relayed to her.

I have renewed faith in human kindness today!

Day of Egg Collection, 9ᵗʰ May 2011:

Everything went really well again, same as before. The fear is of course always in the back of one's mind though. This early morning routine of going up to London is quite daunting.

We are also at the stage where we don't want to keep discussing what we are going through with anyone, for fear of landing all of our emotional baggage upon them. However, when people are that close, you don't even need to say anything…they just know.

Both of our parents have had tears over this or at least been very upset, which is hard.

12ᵗʰ May 2011, Results from Egg Collection:

They took seven follicles, and five had eggs in them (follicles don't always necessarily have eggs within them so this is actually a good result). To cut a long story short, three fertilised, and two were then put back at the transfer, as they were the biggest.

25ᵗʰ May 2011: Sadly, we've had another negative pregnancy test after all of this. I can't write much as I am feeling extremely low today.

6ᵗʰ IVF Cycle
16ᵗʰ August 2011, Second Scan:

Today is our second scan of this our 6ᵗʰ IVF cycle.

As nervous as I always am at what the nurses will find, today was actually looking positive. A massive total of eleven follicles were found altogether. For me, that is a good amount. And in addition, the lady scanning me, the sonographer, Alison who we've got to know quite well now, informed me that five of them were looking large and in the lead. This is good news.

19ᵗʰ August 2011:

Third scan today. There's still eleven follicles altogether which is great. All are growing really well too (that will explain my bloated tummy feeling). The nurse that we consulted after the scan to go through my growth chart etc., informed us that it's looking as though the follicles should be ready for egg collection by next Wednesday (today is Friday).

23rd August 2011:

Fourth scan today. So, it has been now confirmed at this stage that I have seven large follicles and four smaller ones. The nurse informed me that the smaller ones can still catch up and can be retrieved and could of course have eggs inside of them. It's also been confirmed that I will be having the procedure Wednesday at 7 a.m.

I'm now sitting at home with our little Siamese cat, Coco, on my lap who I must say has been my salvation. Whenever we've got back from our egg collections or had any nasty news (or are just feeling low about the whole thing), she sits on our laps as if she knows and gives us comfort. They do say Siamese cats 'have a sixth sense'; I'm sure ours does!

14th August 2011:

Today was egg collection day. I've come round from the anaesthetic now and am sitting up in my hospital bed.

I have great news. An enormous twelve eggs were retrieved this time. Not bad considering I was told in our last scan that I had seven large and four small follicles! All has been fine and I've had a quick recovery so far.

Apparently, this is a great result as of course some follicles often don't even have eggs inside of them. And on top of that it looks like one was obviously hiding in the scans so we have more than we had expected.

I'm nervous as always as we now embark on our journey home and await to hear how the embryos will do.

29th August 2011: Day of embryo transfer. So, three embryos made it. One was a grade two, four cell, one was a grade one, two cell, and the third one was a grade one, two cell. (The grading is the quality of the embryo. The cell size is the amount of cells in the structure that increases within hours).

The transfer itself went smoothly again. The lead up to these transfers is so nerve wracking though. From an emotional point of view, you brace yourself in case you arrive at the hospital and your embryos have taken a turn for the worse or arrested, as literally every minute counts.

On arrival, greeted by the embryologist, doctor and nurse we were informed that since they had done their routine check on the embryos that morning they had again increased in size and quality. One area they study is the outer shell called the zona pellucida, and in our case it was apparently looking 'ready to hatch' which was great news.

So we are now off for the scary two week wait before testing. We have decided to take a break with my mother to Spain which we hope will help with this rather torturous time.

9ᵗʰ September 2011:

We are in Spain. We were hoping that the change of location may improve our chances on this two week wait.

Well, I can't believe that I am actually typing these words. The digital home pregnancy test that I did today said 'pregnant 1–2 weeks'! Paul and I looked at it together to see the result. Then, we looked again and again, checking it over and over, both absolutely elated, shocked and scared all at the same time. Later that morning, we couldn't help but go to see my mother in her bedroom and tell her our news! We were all so overjoyed, but nervous at the same time and in disbelief.

Paul and I still kept looking at the little digital stick and hoping it was right.

Later that day when we were out for lunch, my mother ordered a bottle of Champagne – of course, I was only allowed a sip for the toast!

Later that afternoon:

I have just suffered some slight stomach cramps. But we are just hoping that it is normal early pregnancy symptoms, as we are so happy to see 'pregnant' on our test.

We are so happy! This is the day we had always dreamed of.

12ᵗʰ September 2011:

The same afternoon as the positive test, I unfortunately suffered a lot of heavy bleeding after the stomach cramps. It's been very upsetting and scary.

We went to a Spanish hospital nearby and, under instruction from Dr Michael Dooley on the phone today, we requested a blood test for beta hCG (human chorionic gonadotropin). This is the hormone that reveals if you are pregnant or not. It came back as 64 mIU/ml (at 3 weeks it should be around 5–50 mIU/ml as a guide). So it's not bad, but I've continued bleeding for a further 3 days. Feeling quite lost and don't know what to think. It was difficult explaining to the doctors at the Spanish hospital that this is an IVF pregnancy too since they didn't speak much English (and we don't speak Spanish).

This is such a horrible feeling. It's as though I have a time bomb inside of me and I feel as though I am walking on egg shells. Please let this all be OK…

FACT BOX:

HCG blood test- HCG stands for human chorionic gonadotropin. HCG is a hormone produced by the body during pregnancy. Once a pregnancy has been established, HCG will increase every 72 hours (from 11 days after conception). It will reach its peak measurement at about 11 weeks pregnant.

When a miscarriage occurs, the difficult part is predicting if the pregnancy has vanished or not, since HCG can continue increasing for days afterwards tricking you in to thinking that you may still be pregnant. After a few days to a week, the results will start to plummet so regular HCG blood tests are recommended.

13ᵗʰ September 2011:

Back in the UK, today we have had my hCG blood test done again to check whether it was going up or not. Basically, if you are losing a pregnancy it comes down. This is terrifying.

We've just received the call from the hospital. It was 303! We are so happy…albeit cautiously so. The nurse on the phone said I am four and a half weeks pregnant. We are absolutely elated.

I'm having a 'pregnancy' scan done at The Lister next week and may get another hCG blood test done tomorrow to rest our minds (I hope).

14ᵗʰ September 2011:

I had the blood test and result today, and phew it is 667 mIU/ml…we can sigh with relief. The figure is clearly going up which is great news and positive. The nurse that called me with the results said everything is fine and that bleeding does happen in healthy pregnancies often. Mind you, I haven't had bleeding for a few days now which is a relief.

We are both so, so, so happy.

18ᵗʰ September 2011, (morning):

An, almost black, bleed has started again today. So very worried. Staying in bed today as I am too scared to move. Our pregnancy scan is in four days' time. Not sure we can wait that long.

18ᵗʰ September 2011, (Afternoon):

Saw a Doctor at our local accident and emergency hospital, The Royal Sussex County, as Dr Michael Dooley recommended I call them to ask if they can scan me since it is a weekend. Why do these things always happen over a weekend?

The doctor we saw there, by his own admission, wasn't that knowledgeable about either IVF or, surprisingly, pregnancy. I found myself giving him information again and again and trying to almost give him a quick lesson in what IVF entailed. It was very hard, and just added to the strain we were feeling.

He then did a pregnancy test in front of us both. Negative.

We are both in utter despair. He did say it could be that I had only been to the toilet 20 minutes beforehand as I didn't know that I would be doing a pregnancy test. So the long and short is that we are having a scan and blood test done at our local hospital tomorrow in the Early Pregnancy Unit.

We can't believe that in a large hospital like this, no one could scan me simply because it was a weekend. Apparently, there was no one on duty who could operate a pregnancy scan. It's a disgrace really in this day and age. This to us is an emergency.

So we are now sent home to worry for the night.

19th September 2011, (Morning):

I took a digital pregnancy test at home this morning which once again said 'pregnant 1–2 weeks' to our amazement. I'm going for the scan and HCG blood test today, so we will have a clearer picture afterwards I'm sure.

I'm so nervous that I can't even put it in to words.

19th September 2011, (afternoon):

So we went to the Early Pregnancy Unit in our local hospital. It's a very old fashioned tiny unit with a postage stamp size waiting area of couples squashed together. You only go here when there are problems, so it's not a nice place to visit.

After a nerve-wracking wait, we were taken in to a room for the scan. The nurse spent a while looking over my tummy, then announced the words we had both dreaded, "I'm afraid there is no obvious sign of a pregnancy anymore."

20th September 2011: The day after that terrible scan.

We are feeling shell shocked and very sad. Both have shed many tears.

Also aware that we are both getting angry with the situation today; we are only human. The anger is just another emotion that I guess we have to go through. I spoke to Mr Michael Dooley today who advised us not to attempt any more IVF cycles until after Christmas. He said we need 'to heal in every way and mourn our loss now'. When I asked, he also informed me that our chances of falling pregnant naturally would be lower after a miscarriage. No good news basically.

Feel hopeless. It is currently my magazine deadline week also. My right hand lady, Mo, has been my rock as always. She's also a friend and so probably senses something is wrong.

I'm trying to chase editorial and adverts, while also driving my sales team forward. I won't lie and say it's the best day!

I guess at least focusing on my work helps take my mind away from this pain though, so I'm just plunging myself in to it.

Only a few close people know what's just happened. Feel exhausted physically…and so shattered in every way.

21st September 2011 (morning): This is so hard, getting through my deadline, being in my office, and going through this. I have also suffered more bleeding today…and some pain. Feeling even lower emotionally today too.

I feel the tears on my cheeks whenever I am alone, unaware that I am even crying until I feel them.

21st September 2011 (afternoon): The bleeding has become much heavier now. I now know that this is the miscarriage setting in. I can also feel painful cramps in my abdomen. Emotionally, it's so hard having these physical reminders.

4th October 2011: Paul is not well. Last night he came home from the gym, ate his dinner and then about 30 minutes later had sudden tummy pains and was doubled up in acute pain very quickly. Having spoken to his doctor first, I was instructed to call an ambulance. He was in excruciating pain, shaking and had sweats; it came from nowhere. Very frightening. I thought it must be something he ate; my cooking!

It was later discovered he had a kidney stone. Unfortunately, it apparently wasn't a 'normal' one either, it was 'star shaped' making it even more painful, poor thing. Back at hospital now for his scan…due to its shape, the kidney stone has become dislodged. What a two weeks it's been for us so far! He'll have to have a small operation to remove it, but they are keeping him in hospital until then. Looks like it'll be next week! So on top of what we are going through, we are now separated with Paul at hospital and me at home for a week. Oh well, I am sure we will laugh at all of this one day!

7th IVF Cycle

5th December 2011:

Paul's operation went well. However, it wasn't pleasant for him to say the least; he had to be awake too. Think he's a bit disturbed by it, poor thing!

Having had a break from IVF after all of our recent events, we decided (yet again) that we both really want to keep going.

The funny thing is, that you worry that someday one of you will decide 'enough is enough'. And that would be completely understandable, because this situation to be honest is hellish.

However, somehow, Paul and I want to keep going. Hearing myself say that even sounds a bit crazy. I almost feel embarrassed at how much we are both yearning for a baby together to love and cherish. But my heart really does ache when I consider that we may not succeed. So, the only thing within our power (as we are in the 'unexplained' category) is to keep going with IVF! Obviously, we still hope it may happen 'naturally' so yes, we sure have fun 'trying'!

So here we are about to embark on cycle number seven. Today I had the first scan, which already is showing nine follicles which is good. It feels odd being 'back in the saddle again' so to be speak. But I take a deep breath and just pray it works this time. It's always a gamble. But then, like gambling, there's always a chance we could win!

8th December 2011:

Today was the second scan. Ten follicles are showing altogether! Seven are large. This is a good result so far for us. We always keep positive, and this result certainly helps keep that momentum going.

I've been told by the nurse looking at my chart of the size of the follicles that egg collection for me may be next Wednesday. The only problem with this is that it would be the same day as my magazine deadline. Panic. I will now have to move things around at work. Fortunately, moving a deadline to a later date helps our sales team by giving them extra time for sales. However, the printers may not be able to accommodate it and in addition, it will shorten the subsequent month which is not ideal at this time of the year (approaching the shorter month of Christmas). I will first need to speak to our printers.

I'm also quite stressed as it is the festive season and I feel quite behind workwise/everything wise as we all do this time of the year. I love to always be ahead in what I am doing. Maybe I am just over-panicking though.

10th December 2011:

Feeling very bloated now. Think they'll confirm for me tomorrow when egg collection is definitely due to be booked in.

13th December 2011:

Third scan: There's only seven follicles now. The nurse's say that's still good and it's normal for some to sometimes drop away. I can't help but feel low though. I'm so worried it won't work now after coming this far! Feel quite down.

I think IVF clinics should coach the partners of the women going through IVF on how to look after us 'pin cushions/incubators'…just explaining to our partners that we need some rest could make a huge difference. But then, on the other hand, I do read about some partners who are worried sick so maybe the clinics feel they shouldn't worry them even more? Everyone is different. In our case, I think Paul is putting on an act of 'you're fine' to make me psychologically feel better, which I can totally understand.

Incidentally, for any partners reading this, all we want is a cuddle and to be told how great we are doing at this stage (even simple things like doing dinner for us women at this time or the odd cup of tea also means so much).

When you reach this milestone in a fertility cycle, it's as if you've trained for the Olympics. You've geared your body up, you've emotionally pushed yourself to the limit and told yourself 'you can do it'. So now, you need the applauding crowd. It's actually quite an emotional stage for the woman at this point, but also extremely tiring and nerve wracking (in fact, so physically tiring I cannot put it in to words).

14th December 2011:

I had another scan today. The seven are still looking great thankfully.

As with all scan appointments, you have to have a blood test done as well to check that the hormone levels are correlating well with the follicles growth size. This morning I had a call from the clinic to say that my blood test from yesterday shows I am 'bordering ready' now, so I have had to go back again today. The good news is that everything is looking fine, with the seven large follicles still growing.

The clinic are booking me in for egg collection the day after tomorrow. That means it's all systems go now with three injections tonight.

It's getting hard now as my tummy is very bruised. I am literally injecting in to bruises and hard muscle. I keep telling myself that people go through far worse! It does hurt though. I just bite my lip and do it. The pain I can deal with. It's when I'm feeling emotional while injecting that I find it the hardest. For some reason, when I am feeling upset and inject, the pain increases.

But thankfully after tonight, there will be no more injections or medications. Hurray, that's an amazing feeling.

Although, the NK Cells blood test did flag up that I have 'slightly raised levels'. Therefore, I will be taking the steroid, Prednisolone from now on (but it's only a tablet).

I'm getting nervous now about the egg collection. Being our 7th attempt, I feel there's so much riding on this.

It never gets easier.

15ᵗʰ December 2011:

Egg Collection day: So, I've had it done. Feeling fine again afterwards, which is largely due to the wonderful anaesthetist and surgeon. There are such nice people here at The Lister; our male nurse has such a kind and sunny persona which makes such a difference to the whole experience. We had the BBC News on the television when he entered our room. He started chatting to us about various topics on there, followed by offering me more pillows (and 'anything else' that would make me feel more comfortable). You can sense genuine care when you come across it.

Anyway, they managed to retrieve six eggs out of the seven follicles which is OK (although they tell me 'this is great').

As always, I am just praying it will all be OK this time and I fall pregnant with that much-wanted baby…feel we need some luck with this. But I feel more anxious than ever for this to work, for us to welcome our own baby in to the world (and give Niomi a little sibling).

17th December 2011:

Embryo transfer day: It was a two-day transfer so we were both disappointed. Basically, transfers are usually up to six days later. The later the better as it shows that there was more of a choice for selection; some embryos die off. The fittest will survive.

Five out of the six embryos were able to be injected. Three were no good, so two were left.

We both felt down. However, when we got to the hospital they gave us the amazing news that the two embryos were the best quality we have had so far. Both were grade 1 (as good as it gets). One a four cell and one a five cell which is very good.

I felt so nervous throughout the procedure. I couldn't stop my legs shaking which has never happened before (very embarrassing). All the staff doing the procedure were amazingly nice to me and said how much we deserve this to happen. I feel quite emotional now. We are on the train home. I feel like I need a good cry (but then I worry this will damage our chances. So I must try to be upbeat and strong with this little thing inside me now, and so instead smile).

28th December 2011:

We actually managed to enjoy Christmas and wore happy faces. We are not putting on an act though. On the contrary, it helps to be happy with everyone and wear brave faces (plus I absolutely love Christmas)!

In fact, Christmas Day was one example of us going with the flow pushing our current situation to the back of our minds. I am forever proud of Paul, but this time in particular. Having my gorgeous little niece at my mother's house on Christmas Day, my mother decided to get down the Santa outfit from her attic. But, none of the men in the house would wear it, all feeling a bit tired and full of festive food by then! Paul being Paul, was kind enough to don the (rather dusty old) suit at my mother's request and ring the doorbell to greet my little niece. How proud was I of this man! At the moment we don't know if we can have a child together, but there he is playing Santa for the kids. We've always said we will carry on regardless, and what I mean by that is, we agreed we mustn't be selfish and allow this situation to prevent us from any potentially difficult situations. Life must still be fun.

No one knows of course what we are going through this week, not even our parents this time. We didn't want to cause worry for anyone over Christmas.

It's also now the night before we test; I'm feeling very anxious and worried.

This is the hardest and most emotional part of our journey now by far. No one can understand this feeling unless they've been through it. The last few days I have suffered similar period-like symptoms on and off with small aches here and there. Some days I am so sure it hasn't worked that I am tearful. But then, I remind myself that the embryologist said the two that they put back at two days were our best quality so far. And in our scans, my lining had the magical three layers and shape that I was told is what they always want for a good embedding of embryos…here's to anxiously hoping, but terrifyingly scared. Please God, let this be our time.

29th December 2011:

The test was negative. Distraught and confused, and I know you may wonder why, but we're in shock. Every negative brings up more questions and sheer panic in our minds. Why is this happening to us? We have sent an email to our consultant doctor, Mr Raef Faris and also to Mr Michael Dooley to give them the result and also get their input on the situation.

All I can say is, we are so very sad today…

30th December 2011:

The day after our negative test:
Feeling like I've now hit rock bottom. I can't stop crying.

Beginning to realise there may be no hope now. I then feel very selfish too for saying that, as I know people are going through far worse in the world than this.

However, I feel desperately sad. This is such a testing time for us as a couple too. We've had tears, guilt, despair and anger all in the last 24 hours. I have tears as I type this.

The plan now is to have some more blood tests done on the NHS as recommended by Dr Raef Faris and Mr Michael Dooley: thyroid, cholesterol, AMH, FSH, full blood count, AMH and oestradiol, and anti-protein C resistance. There was even talk of whether I should have a mammogram!

Meanwhile, I have quite a few events in the diary now that I must attend to represent our magazine. I've got used to taking a deep breath and walking in with a brave face (it reminds me of when I used to attend such events alone as a freelance journalist in my early days in this career)! Paul is exactly the same, I can tell.

9th January 2012:

To add to our stresses, today we've had a tribunal with a former member of our staff, a manager, who left our restaurant business unexpectedly after arguing with other members of our team. We now have to pay £27k to them for 'unfair dismissal' (even though, like I say, they walked out on us unannounced leaving the business in the lurch. It was almost impossible to demonstrate this as it was his word against ours). They worked for us for only 18 months. We've since learnt this person has done this with previous employers too, subsequently suing them, but that information is not allowed to be disclosed during a tribunal. What a crazy world we live in. But that's the difference when it's your own business, as oppose to if it was a job that we could just walk away from. Our heart and souls and finances are our businesses.

So now, all we can think about is how much that £27k would have gone towards on our procedures? Yes, we feel beaten down today.

To summarise, we've had seven IVFs, one miscarriage, Paul's had a kidney stone operation, (and now we've been sued)…oh, and Paul has just told me he is at hospital tomorrow as he has had some worrying symptoms. And on a very sad note, a very close and dear friend of ours is currently very ill.

It can be hard at times like these periods in life, to remain focused on what we are going through with the IVF.

Anyway, I had the blood tests and results. The only one that flagged up a change is the thyroid one. I am very borderline low.

There is nowadays evidence to suggest that being slightly low with thyroid activity can actually be a hindrance to women falling pregnant. Therefore, I have been sent to see a specialist in this area, Professor Lesley, who is also based at The Lister hospital.

The meeting went very well and he confirmed that when thyroid hormones drop too low (hypothyroidism) it can adversely affect fertility and even be a cause for miscarriage.

Therefore he has prescribed 25 mcg (a very minimal dose) of Levothyroxine once a day indefinitely. He also informed me that this drug does not in any way negatively affect falling pregnant and that it is still safe to continue taking during pregnancy.

And Paul's visit to the doctor? Well, it was quite a funny one in the end. He had been passing red urine. Naturally, we were alarmed. However, we soon discovered from the doctor that Paul's great love of *beetroot* was the actual reason. It can dye your urine. We did laugh lots when we found out!

FACT BOX:

Hypothyroidism- This is when the thyroid produces less thyroid hormone than it should which causes the metabolism to run too slow. This is also called myxoedema or an underactive thyroid. It may also be called Hashimoto's disease.

Hypothyroidism can affect fertility by discouraging the body to produce so many eggs each month, as well as other factors required for a successful pregnancy to occur.

11ᵗʰ January 2012:

Today we had a re-group meeting with Dr Michael Dooley. It seemed to go well at the time, but now I find myself feeling extremely low about it all now I'm at home. The main conclusion of the meeting was that there is no reason why it's not happening for us. We are also having more bloods taken – I had eight today alone. And there's more to come. At the end of the meeting, Mr Dooley said that if after two more IVFs we fail, we should consider donor eggs...this has made me more distraught than words could ever say. I just can't imagine carrying someone else's baby inside me. While I respect anyone that can and will carry donated eggs, for me it is a personal decision that I feel I can't; the result would be half my husband and half another woman. It would just feel odd. Paul has also asked me if I would consider this. In his opinion, he says he would prefer a child that is at least half his rather than none at all. Why am I being handed such a cruel cross to bear? And what's also making me feel worse now is that the three of us in the meeting had the discussion about my age again... I am now 37. Time has now moved on. Then Mr Dooley pointed out that it 'might' work using, for example, a 22-year-old's eggs. Hearing the two men discuss my age like this made me feel like a redundant old machine... I hate this so much. I am struggling. But I also appreciate that I am probably being over-emotional at the moment. Of course, they don't mean to hurt me at all. It is just a conversation that we have to have.

8ᵗʰ IVF Cycle

5ᵗʰ May 2012:

So we've decided after deliberating and discussing the options with Dr Raef Faris and Dr Michael Dooley that we will go ahead with another IVF. However, the main conclusion has been that we should now try ICSI again as opposed to standard IVF. Yes, it's a bit more expensive by the best part of £1000, but hearing that it increases our chances we are of course willing to give ICSI another go (we tried it in an earlier cycle).

However, today on our way to The Lister for an appointment we saw the front page of the Daily Mail newspaper stating 'IVF ICSI causes birth defects.' Obviously, we are now completely alarmed by this statement so we have asked if we can discuss this with someone. Our nurse is finding out if anyone is available to talk to us.

6th May 2012:

Yesterday, after we had made our fears clear having seen the Daily Mail article on ICSI, the head embryologist at The Lister, Safira, came to see us in a private room. She was completely thorough and sympathetic when explaining to us the details of that report. She told us how while a study was indeed conducted by 'a professor', it was not carried out by the HFEA (Human Fertilisation and Embryology Authority). Secondly, the professor only looked at couples who already had an increased risk of giving birth to a child with birth defects due to their own family history.

She was extremely knowledgeable and reassured us that even if her own 'sister needed ICSI' she would definitely recommend her to try it.

Safira has completely put us both at ease now and we are sure what we are doing is the correct thing. Neither of us have a family history, thankfully, and all of our blood tests are showing up as normal so far.

Safira then asked us how we were and what stage we were at. She was so informative yet kind and not at all patronising about our situation or about how many IVFs we have had.

We are now starting to realise that although people always assume the hospital/clinic and doctor are key to you falling pregnant during IVF, it is equally as vital to have an excellent embryologist working on your results and an up-to-date high tech laboratory. What goes on behind the scenes in those laboratories is of the utmost importance in this game. Fortunately, The Lister has a state-of-the-art laboratory. And with us now knowing Safira, who is leading the team there, we feel even more confident.

24th May 2012:

I didn't write about this cycle until now as to be honest, I did feel quite apprehensive about the whole thing. I just couldn't bring myself to write about it. However, today I had my egg collection and they managed to retrieve eight eggs out of nine follicles. The staff was amazing as always. Safira (the head of embryology) visited us afterwards to give us an inside view of how everything went. She is amazing and so kind to give us this hands on approach. She said that she is going to personally be watching our embryos from now on.

Physically, I'm OK again this time, just bleeding (like a period) which hasn't happened before and have slight cramps and feel worn out which is all apparently normal. We will get the call in the morning to say how the embryos are progressing.

25th May 2012:

Safira called us to say that five out of eight eggs were injected (in other words were viable for injecting). This is good.

As a result, four have now fertilised.

27th May 2012:

Day of the embryo transfer:

I had two embryos put back today, which is a day three transfer.

One is a grade one using a grade one sperm, and is a five cell.

The other one is a grade three, this is an eight cell.

Now it's over to the two week wait.

Fingers crossed as always!

6th June 2012:

A small amount of brown discharge has appeared. I'm so worried.

I have slight tummy cramps and my abdomen feels how is does when a period is arriving.

We've also been under more stress lately with our businesses, so I'm very worried the stress has affected this cycle and it hasn't worked or that it has affected it if it has – desperately anxious. Can't stop feeling down now as I think something has gone wrong.

I can't talk to Paul as it makes it feel more real and it will only upset and worry him too. But I am also not going to talk to anyone else about it. That's the trouble with this infertility world; through your own fault you end up feeling quite alone in this situation.

8th June 2012:

Today we did the pregnancy test, which sadly said negative.

We are desperately sad and in that complete shell-shock mode again.

I spent the day indoors mourning this failed cycle with Paul.

On the physical side of things, there is still only slight brown discharge. I'm very confused about that, but I guess we are just still hoping.

8th June 2012:

Spoke to Dr Raef Faris last night. He advised us to do another pregnancy test this morning but we were too sad to see another 'negative' so we decided to wait for the dreaded period to arrive and let nature tell us instead.

I've had meetings all day, and low and behold it arrived halfway through.

I've been in an awful lot of pain. I don't usually get period pains. Now worried it may have been another miscarriage, as it feels similar.

We both feel quite distraught.

Even with all our other problems going on in other areas, we've said if I was pregnant everything would simply pale in to insignificance.

We just don't know which direction our lives are going in now, and that's the trouble with this terrible journey for any couple going through it.

We've decided we can't currently afford another IVF cycle, but maybe that's a good thing as maybe we can't emotionally either. All of our businesses are experiencing testing times in this recession. And this is starting to feel as if we are pouring money down the drain.

3rd July 2012:

It has been an awful time. I have suffered extraordinary events since my last entry.

The bleeding (from what we thought was my period for a few days) stopped as normal. Then a week later started again as light brown spotting which lasted for a few days.

Eventually, we thought I should call someone for advice. It must be a hormone problem I began to think. I couldn't get hold of anyone at that particular time at The Lister so I decided to call Mr Dooley.

He requested that I do a pregnancy test. I asked him, "Why," and I explained that I had already done one weeks ago that was negative.

But he simply said, "Please do another one as quickly as you can and then we will go from there. Call me as soon as you've done it."

Confused, I jumped in to my car and went to the local shops, bought one, I didn't even tell Paul as he was in a meeting and I didn't see the need to bother him.

I stood knowing it would say negative again…but to my utter amazement, it said 'pregnant'! I didn't know whether to be elated or sad. What was going on? I quickly called Mr Dooley who calmly said, "Please don't get excited. I want you to now call The Lister and request a blood test and scan today to rule out anything nasty." Nasty? I wasn't sure what he meant. Then I realised, obviously another miscarriage.

Staying calm, I called The Lister and spoke to a nurse who said yes they would do a blood test today but it was too early for a scan.

I then called Paul. Like me, he was completely confused by this. Why would the test say negative a few weeks ago followed by a period, and now one says 'pregnant'? We felt a bit numb.

Paul and I went for the hCG blood test at The Lister. The nurse taking it said it may be a miscarriage or could just be a normal bleed in an early pregnancy. We hoped and prayed for the latter and that all would be OK. However, we still couldn't get our heads around the fact that I WAS actually officially pregnant!

The blood test result came through that afternoon when we were at home and confirmed that, yes, I was indeed pregnant.

I asked the nurse who gave me the result over the phone what could the bleeding be then? She said, "It could be any number of things, but just be happy. You're pregnant. Relax now," and then she congratulated me.

I was not happy though for some reason. My instinct kept telling me that this light bleeding I was suffering was wrong.

I called Mr Dooley who immediately said, "Please don't get your hopes up by the blood test result or the pregnancy test result."

I replied, "I'm not." He then informed me that we needed to eliminate anything 'nasty' that could be going on inside of me. I asked what he meant and he said 'an ectopic pregnancy' was his main concern but I mustn't worry myself too much as this was unusual and I'd be very unlucky indeed. He instructed me to call The Lister again and request a scan for that same afternoon.

So I called The Lister again that same day (20th June 2012) and requested a scan. The nurse I spoke to suggested I wait two days until Friday when they had their next available appointments. However, it sounds silly, but I was meant to be attending Ascot Ladies Day in the Royal Enclosure the following day (and it would be Niomi's first time) and so I kept thinking to myself I wanted to be able to relax there with peace of mind. I didn't want to be worrying about what the bleeding was all day.

So it was with that in mind, thank goodness, that made me push the nurse for a scan that same afternoon (just as Michael Dooley had also requested me to do).

I later discovered that that decision saved my life. Thank goodness for Ascot really. But especially, Dr Michael Dooley!

I said to Paul, as he had so much work on, not to worry about coming back to The Lister that day with me for the scan. I was convinced I would be fine and we had already travelled up to London once that day (in the boiling hot sunshine). Why should we *both* keep going through this torture?

I was taken through for my scan by our usual lovely sonographer, Alison. Almost immediately as she started the scan, probably to put me quickly out of my misery, she carefully informed me that 'sadly there was clearly a pregnancy inside the left fallopian tube; an ectopic pregnancy'.

My heart sank. I probably went in to shock. In fact, I know I did. And when I go in to shock, I go in to autopilot 'cope mode'. Alison also looked sad, as having seen Paul and me so many times, I could see in her face that she knew what a blow this would be for us. I recall her saying to me, "Ectopic pregnancies are the cruellest test of all during infertility." My mind was swirling. I started shaking. What did this now mean? I asked her naïvely if there was any way that they could retrieve the fetus and then place it in to my uterus. She said, "Sadly, no one's discovered a way of doing that yet. If only there was a way. I am so sorry."

She then left me alone in her office and said to use her private landline to call Paul. I said I can use my mobile, but as she left the room, she gently said, "Just take your time on my landline." I sensed how sad she was too. What I now know is, being in the profession she is in, Alison would have been very aware what I would now have to endure and what the consequences meant.

It was devastating telling Paul. There was no nice way of telling him. The facts were the facts. I could hear the panic in his voice. I didn't know what happened now or where I should go? Do I have an operation now?

Alison returned to take me to the waiting area where I would be called to see a doctor who would explain everything. It felt like forever sitting there alone watching the world going normally by. I kept shaking from the shock setting in.

Next, my mother called me as she hadn't been able to get hold of me all day; I explained to her what had happened. I did not want to panic her, I said I was coping just fine.

I had not met the doctor before who called me through. He was kind and sympathetic, and explained to me that the simplest way to imagine it is that the embryo is like a car that has entered in to a parking space that it shouldn't have; the opening of the fallopian tube. This is very rare. Apparently, embryos bounce around for a few days before they settle or 'park' somewhere in the uterus where they will eventually grow. And so in our unfortunate circumstance, it had gone in to and landed in my left fallopian tube and there it carried on growing. This can happen with IVF or naturally. He explained that it was simply pure bad luck.

He then went on to explain that the only option was surgery. As the fallopian tube had not ruptured, and he felt sure that it wouldn't, he said surgery could take place in the morning.

I had the choice of having the operation either done at The Lister or at the nearby Chelsea and Westminster Hospital, which of course being an NHS hospital would be free and save us thousands of pounds. He reassured me of how good The Chelsea and Westminster Hospital was having trained there himself and so I agreed to have the operation there. Also, as there was an A&E department there if needed, it made sense. Hopefully, all they would have to do was remove the embryo, not the tube though.

I returned to the waiting room and called Paul and my mother again to update them. They both said that they would meet me there at The Chelsea and Westminster with my overnight bag. Paul was in a state of shock, I could tell. I hated hearing him like this. He was flapping and his voice was breaking. My mum sounded the same. I had to keep them together and keep everything on an even keel. Paul was calling Niomi for me as I was then informed that I had to arrange my transport to the hospital quickly. I later discovered from her that she was in a shopping centre when he called her and that she burst in to tears and nearly fainted. I felt so terrible hearing this. I initially thought and hoped that I could go through this whole experience without having to tell and worry her.

I travelled to the hospital by taxi. The doctor from The Lister told me that when I arrive at the Chelsea and Westminster Hospital to hand them my file at A&E and that I would then be seen straightway as my doctor knew the surgeon that would look after me and he had called him in advance.

Shortly after I arrived, Paul and my mother did too.

I handed over the file and explained the urgency and that I had been told to see someone immediately, but I was told to sit and wait. We waited 40 minutes. It felt like days.

I was eventually called through where I was checked in a cubicle by a nurse for everything including diabetes and anaemia, but nothing to do with the ectopic pregnancy that was inside of me.

By now, what was happening to me started to sink in (albeit in a surreal way). I asked if I could have the operation that same evening to get it over and done with; but was informed it was not possible as it was getting late now and they did not like to operate 'in the dark'. It would be in the morning.

Eventually, I was taken up to see the surgeon for a check over. I think he was surprised that I was not in any pain and that I turned down the painkillers. I'd been avoiding pain killers for so long now due to the infertility, I think I had got used to it.

I also asked him if I could have the operation that night; I just couldn't imagine sleeping with this inside me feeling like this. All I felt was a slight tingling or trickling in my tummy now but I wasn't sure if I was imagining it.

The doctor said he'd like to do a quick scan then before he departed for the night to see where the embryo was exactly.

Paul and my mother were in the room as he scanned me. The worst part for me at that moment was seeing their distressed faces. I kept reassuring them I was fine and smiling calmly. But they were both grey faced and sad; I felt terrible for them watching me like this. All I could do was repeat that I was fine and in excellent hands.

Instantly, upon scanning me, the doctor said quite loudly to the nurse and to us that 'the fallopian tube had unfortunately now ruptured' and that I had internal bleeding; he explained this was now an 'emergency situation with 40 minutes to stop it'. Apparently, my uterus cavity was quickly filling with blood.

I was going to be operated on as soon as possible after all.

He pressed a button on the wall and suddenly people came running in prepping me for the operation. One was suddenly taking off my nail varnish with remover while the anaesthetist was checking my medical history asking me necessary questions very quickly.

My mother and Paul went out to the waiting area for a few minutes. It must have been terrible for them. Apparently, one of the doctors apologised to them both for what they were about to hear as he picked up the phone; he was shouting to someone words to the effect that they had 'a lady requiring emergency surgery, get theatre ready now...I mean NOW! We could lose her'!

Meanwhile, I felt calm (bearing in mind I didn't know about the above conversation until afterwards), and just wanted this done quickly. I also sensed that I was in extremely capable and safe hands, which helped hugely.

Saying bye to Paul and my mother as I went through to theatre though, was really horrible as I could see how worried they were. I told them to go over the road to 'Carluccio's' for dinner and that I'd be fine. I also told them to call Niomi and inform her that I was fine and loved her very much, and that I really wanted her to still go to Ascot the next day as she (and her boyfriend Marcus) had been so excited and she had her outfit and hat all ready. In fact, I kept telling them that I was adamant she must still go.

There wasn't time to get me a wheelchair or porter with a bed, so a nurse walked me to theatre as they wanted to get me there as soon as possible; the surgeon commented with a smile that he had never before seen a 'walk in' in his surgery, which amused me.

I sat in the corridor with the nurse just outside of the main operating theatre while they prepared it, and we chatted about everyday things for a few minutes making small talk; it was all very surreal.

Then they called me through.

21st June 2012, (Going Back to after the Events of 20th June):

I woke up on a ward (minus a fallopian tube, as it could not be saved sadly).

I believe my mother and Paul visited me briefly (in the night). Niomi was also brought up to see me by my older brother,

Jai, around midnight, but my mother and Paul explained I was asleep and so they all returned in the same car to Sussex together. My poor brother had driven all the way up to London during the night to only turn around and go back again.

In the morning, I remember lying in my hospital bed. For some reason, I was in a room of ladies who were mostly pregnant with complications or had just given birth to their babies. I could hear them all chatting around me about their babies and pregnancies – all minor issues, so they were all quite happy and comparing pregnancy and baby notes. It was so hard to lie in bed and hear their banter.

I now had stitches in three places (under my belly button, and in two circles either side of my pelvic area near my hips; one larger where the tube was removed). Overall, they were actually surprisingly small as it was done by key-hole surgery. Amazing really, for such a serious operation.

I was offered painkillers several times in hospital but still declined. I actually didn't feel much pain at this stage. I think that perhaps my body goes numb when pain is that bad (I actually never had pain relief when I gave birth to Niomi, other than gas and air). And also, as I mentioned earlier, when you go through infertility for a long period of time I think you start to get used to declining any form of unnecessary medication (for example, there are theories that Ibuprofen can cause miscarriage when taken even months before a pregnancy occurs).

My father was the first person in the morning to call me at the hospital; the nurse brought the phone to me. He was so concerned. It was horrible hearing all the upset in everyone's voices. I felt so guilty putting them all through this worry.

But I tried my best to cheerily reassure everyone that I was OK.

I told the nurses and Sister on the ward that I really would like to go home that afternoon. After each IVF operation, I always wanted to just recover in my own home, and this was no different.

They checked me over thoroughly, and explained that it would take about 3–6 months to fully recover and that maybe another night or two in hospital would be wise. But I assured them I would be fine at home. The surgeon who had operated on me also visited me; I couldn't thank him enough (I later followed this up with a thank-you letter, once over time, this episode had sunk in and that I'd been told he had actually saved my life).

Over the coming weeks and months, and even now to a certain extent, it dawned on both Paul and I how lucky I was; the thought that I could have been in bed asleep when this all happened for example didn't bear worth thinking about (we were informed that I wouldn't have known about the internal bleeding). Or even if I had been at Ascot after all, fainting and us not knowing what was wrong. Apparently, I could have just collapsed and then who knows what would have followed. The doctor at the hospital said that I had approximately 30 minutes from the internal bleeding. This was a very lucky escape. So I had to focus on the positive of being 'lucky'. And I didn't believe in wallowing in 'oh that could have been awful…'

So now, my recovery began. I was home with one less fallopian tube…but alive.

Continuation of Events:

People around me were all so kind. I had many good wishes sent to me along with cards and flowers.

A couple of weeks later, we decided to go to my mother and stepfather's flat in Spain for a few days' recovery once I was a bit more mobile. Respite in the sun was a lovely thought.

Getting there was not easy though. In fact, I needed a wheelchair at the airport as I was still not quite steady on my feet and still had the stiches in my tummy. But once I was there, being away from everything in the UK and just having some warmth on my body, really helped. I still couldn't believe what had happened. As with all pregnancies, we always knew there was a minute risk, but still after all we had already gone through, neither of us thought we would also be dealt this card. However, being an optimist, I knew it could have been a lot worse. I had to focus on how lucky I was in the grand scale of things.

But then, we started to think, *could that have been our viable pregnancy*?

The holiday was good, although of course I couldn't swim due to the stitches or go on long walks or such. But then, during all of the little trips that we have taken throughout any IVF cycles, I have not been able to swim (as it can hinder your chances). So really, I am used to that little sacrifice. I even threw caution to the wind with my stitched up tummy in full view on the beach. My thirteen-year-old niece, Arabella, who I adore, was out there too with my mother and stepfather. I was conscious that the stitches could upset her if she saw them.

Fortunately, my bikini bottoms covered one area from everyone's view, while the other two were unfortunately on show. But I don't think you could see unless you were looking deliberately. To be honest, I am also beyond caring what the public on a beach may think, as right now I just need to get better.

An upsetting incident occurred while I was recuperating in Spain when I received a text from someone informing me in a joyous way that they had some happy pregnancy news for me. It was their third pregnancy. I felt hurt, as they knew only too well what I had just gone through with the ectopic pregnancy, and they didn't even ask how I was. I felt it was just insensitive. Nonetheless, I sent a congratulatory message back the following morning. All babies are blessings, as I know only too well. Unfortunately, they responded to my message with anger as they said I had texted them back a congratulations 'too late' (it was the next day). It contained words I'd prefer not to repeat. I didn't respond again, despite more abusive messages coming my way.

There was no reason for my lateness other than I was simply physically worn out and mentally fatigued, and a bit shocked by their insensitivity. You lose track of time when you've been through a physical and emotional trauma. This incident really sent shock waves through me and upset me so much (I think it will for a long time too). But then, so many people have also been so kind to me, so I must focus on that instead. And of course, where there is good there will always be bad, where there is light there will always be dark. Afterwards I was informed that this person may not be in a mentally sound state of mind at the moment. So of course, I must eventually forgive them. However, this episode has really upset me.

I must focus on the good wishes that have been sent my way too at this period in my life by so many caring people.

A few days later:

During our holiday, we had a phone call from a neighbour back in England that they had seen our little cat, (and comforter) Coco, walking past their house injured. I immediately called my parents-in-law who had been popping in each day to feed her (and cuddle her)!

After a few desperate days of them all looking for her and placing posters up in the area and knocking on doors, sadly we then received a phone call when we were at Málaga Airport to return home. It was from Paul's stepfather, John, to say that she had been found in a neighbour's bushes, dead, clearly attacked by another animal.

It may sound odd, especially to non-cat or animal lovers, but we stood at the airport and felt like once again our hearts had been ripped out. We had always said half-heartedly that Coco was our surrogate baby and often said, "What would we do without her." She was like a part of our family to Paul, Niomi and I. Why was life even taking her away from us…especially at this time?

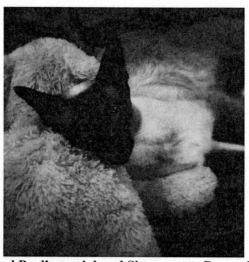

Verity and Paul's much loved Siamese cat, Coco, who sadly went missing at a difficult time for the couple.

9th IVF Cycle

18th September 2012:

The healing process took a while both physically and emotionally.

We visited Dr Raef Faris post ectopic pregnancy, and had it explained to us that having one fallopian tube (or even none) does not actually affect your chances with IVF because the eggs are taken from the ovaries (which I still had both of). The embryos are placed directly in to the uterus during IVF. However, our chances of trying naturally had now been depleted by 35%.

I know a lot of people will be shocked, or even horrified, to know that we could even contemplate doing another round of IVF after all of this, but in a way I think 'not giving up' helped me recover quickly; my fear was always that we would one day have to give up. For as long as we had 'hope' we had to have faith and keep going; we are both optimists after all.

Raef also explained to us, as did Michael Dooley, that this was an extremely unlucky incident to have occurred after all we had been through. They both sounded genuinely surprised, and upset, that this had happened to us.

But stiff upper lipped, and with all the hope we could muster up, we decided to go for another cycle. My mother pleaded with me at this stage to give up. She was understandably worried. But I had to explain, that what had occurred with the ectopic was very rare. As we have been so 'unlucky', there must be some 'luck' coming our way eventually.

Paul's mother, Christine, has also been extremely concerned. We have had a few tears with her by now.

The worry we've caused our mothers is upsetting for us. But at the same time, something keeps telling us not to give up. It's so tough.

So, in this our next cycle, my first scan (before medication) has shown 10 follicles, which is great.

I am still taking my folic acid (which I have since we started trying for a baby). It sounds odd, but even taking that pill each day becomes a chore as you start to think, am I wasting my time? You can become resentful of anything that you have to do in fact.

Meanwhile, on the work front, the ectopic pregnancy experience has really made us both stop and think about our lives, and how short they are. We are investigating selling the magazine. I know if it happens in many ways it will break my heart, but one should never be emotional in business. It is taking up more and more of my time, and the deadlines are tougher than ever with sales going on through to the late evenings nowadays, largely due to the recession. Being in the public eye, without wanting to ward off advertisers, it is a difficult business to market for a sale. So we shall see.

22nd September 2012:

Today, I've had my second scan and the results were seven large follicles with two medium ones which may come through. So all is good so far.

However, I am not sleeping well. I told Alison, our sonographer who said it was probably anxiety with this being our first cycle since the ectopic pregnancy. She fully understood. And I agree with her as last night my mind was wondering with horrible thoughts such as 'what if I'd not been at hospital when it happened', or even imagine if I had been in hospital but asleep in bed as originally planned. Scary.

I also felt very tearful today walking in to The Lister. As I walked up the stairs, I could feel my eyes welling up, but I did not know why. It's probably a mixture of feeling 'here we go again', and the reality of what is still happening to us hitting me again; we are still going through this infertility nightmare. I know that all women (and men) going through this, will know exactly what I mean when I say 'it takes you by surprise'; you can be walking along just fine, and then boom from nowhere you feel yourself crumble.

Mind you, as always, Paul cheered me up in the waiting room. We were chuckling at the fact that our 'file' the doctors and nurses carry every time they see us is about twice as thick as those of all the other patients being called through and 'will probably require a wheelbarrow soon to carry it in'!

24th September 2012:

Today was my third scan for this cycle. Nine large follicles were seen with one smaller one following behind. So one follicle has obviously caught up with the bigger ones, which is great.

I was given the procedure forms as well for egg collection as that was to be on Wednesday (today is Friday). However, I just received a phone call to say it will now be Thursday due to my blood test results this afternoon. Changing the day has made me feel anxious for some reason. I don't know why. Apparently, the doctor who looked at my notes and results this afternoon said that she would prefer to allow the smaller follicles to grow more.

The trouble is, I don't have enough Orgalutran to inject (the drug used to prevent premature ovulation when injecting with Gonal F to stimulate the ovaries) as I only had enough to last until a Wednesday procedure, so I have to travel back to London again tomorrow. Pain. But that is another feature of this IVF game; you have to be able to drop everything and just go. Thank goodness I work for myself. As I've said before, I do feel for people who have to keep explaining to their bosses or taking their holiday time for this (and let's face it, you need those holiday days more than ever when you go through this).

For a while now, I have not been sleeping well. I was very emotional this morning talking to Paul about it all (I had a few tears). This isn't a regular occurrence for me. You get to the stage in this game where you become so tired of trying to be brave, that it can just blurt out. I also can't stop worrying about having another ectopic pregnancy, or such, too. I think that generally tough situations often hit me later. This certainly is…like a brick.

Anyway, I am trying to calm myself down now. Paul meanwhile has coped amazingly well. He plunged himself in to work which is a great medicine in itself. But I can't stop worrying about him too and what's he's really feeling inside.

Meanwhile, we are waiting to hear today if we've sold one of our businesses, our magazine. Although in many ways, it will be a relief as the time feels right, I think these things all add to the emotional rollercoaster that I am on at the moment. I have also loved that magazine with all my heart putting in so much work and effort creating it from scratch, and I love my wonderful team. Unfortunately, the person we are selling our magazine to is not the easiest of people to deal with either which is making the whole process harder and more complicated. I just hope they look after my loyal team!

So now, it's home to do my daily injections. And although I've now done hundreds of the little blighters, I still do struggle a bit with them.

I've now injected in public toilets at weddings (then gone back out on the dance floor!), at theatres and even on an evening in a castle when we went to see a friend of ours sing in a concert! You have to laugh…if only anyone knew.

Paul keeps me going at this stage of the process too with a funny song he has come up with. It's his own version of 'I'm Just a Love Machine' (by The Miracles). He sings to me, "She's just an egg machine," followed by some great seventies' moves dancing! It's good to somehow find humour through all of this…you need it.

27th September 2012:

To cut another long story short, our egg collection was delayed by a day to give the smaller follicles more time to grow.

I am just waiting now to go in to the operating theatre. Same old. And Paul has just gone downstairs to do 'his business', poor thing. He hates this part. He says that walking through the corridor for all of them (the men) is like 'a walk of shame'!

The time is now 08:20 a.m. We woke up at 5 a.m. I'm feeling jaded, hungry (as I can't eat or drink), tired and slightly anxious. Hoping for good numbers.

Post Procedure:

I am back from surgery now and woke up about an hour ago. Everyone took care of me as usual as well as being so professional. They constantly check my every need and don't tire of asking how I am feeling. Even the anaesthetist said to me as I was being put under 'I am sure it'll work this time and we won't see you again'.

They retrieved seven out of nine, as two were too small. The good news is that seven out of seven had eggs inside too (they don't always). Dr Zara who did the procedure this time said this is excellent.

Safira (head of embryology) popped up to see us a she always does now. She agreed that this is an excellent result. Once again, she will be overseeing the sperm and egg grading which is reassuring for us to know.

A Couple of Hours Later:

We are in our room still and we've just had a call from the laboratory downstairs. The man we spoke to said that five out of seven are definitely good to use, two were slightly abnormal. So now, we are down to five. He said that is fine though.

He added that everyone in the laboratory 'is rooting for us'. Safira is going to check everything too.

They'll call us with results tomorrow. So now, we are keeping everything crossed.

We got back to our car at Gatwick Airport car park and unfortunately, the car battery was dead! After the whole early morning expedition (5 a.m.). Paul had forgotten to turn the lights off (or keep them on auto). It's not worth getting upset about these things though (especially after what we've gone through today). I sat quietly in the car while poor Paul sought help. Two guys from the car park arrived quickly with jump leads thank goodness (this is obviously a regular occurrence there). Poor Paul…sometimes I think we worry we are losing our minds through all of this!

30th September 2012:

Three days after egg collection:

I had a call today from Safira to say we're going to have two 'grade one' embryos put back. Hurray. I've been awake all night worrying too so this is great news…so far. We've never had two grade 1's put back!

One is a six cell and one is an eight cell. Safira said she was feeling 'goggle-eyed' from looking through the microscope for so long to select the very best sperm for each egg. We are very lucky indeed. This is why an excellent and caring laboratory team is so important.

30th September 2012:

Day of the embryo transfer:

Our train was delayed! There was an emergency on the train in front of ours and so we were delayed by 40 minutes. We were in such a panic, as we knew that the hospital would get the embryos prepared for our exact time slot and I was worried about their temperature now.

When we finally arrived at the hospital the nurse, embryologist and doctor were all very sympathetic and upbeat saying 'it's really no problem' – phew!

Anyway, the good news is that one embryo had moved on in cell size in just two hours so as I write this I now have on board a seven cell and an eight cell, both grade ones. Emma, today's embryologist, said how very happy she is with them too.

She said in her own words that "it's been horrible for the team watching two lovely people go through such an awful time" and that she really wished us every success. What a kind and sincere thing to say. I shall never forget that. It makes such a difference when you know that you have a team of people backing you up like that. Our doctor today, who put the embryos back, was also lovely. Everything was fine. I joked to Paul how surreal it is that during these procedures we all manage to somehow talk and joke. It's got to be one of the most bizarre rooms to be a fly on the wall! I guess it's the best way to relax ladies in such a horrible situation, and they are really good at doing that. Paul was so kind as always holding my hand and rubbing my brow, and said afterwards that I am such a 'dignified lady'. It made my eyes well up. It sounds silly, but it is one of the many fears you have during this experience that you may lose dignity as a woman.

So now, on to the dreaded two week wait.

11th October 2012:

Update:
The day before the official test day, we decided to test early. It was a big fat negative. Utterly devastated.

Naturally, after all of the effort and upheaval of another few weeks trying like this, we both feel totally deflated and cannot understand what went wrong.

As always with this game, having read your negative result, you then have to carry on with the normality of life, whether that be work, shopping or just going about appointments. Every minute I find my mind is haunted by that negative result again. Walking along or driving I play it round and round in my mind questioning if there was anything I could have done differently.

But that is the challenge, you never actually know why an embryo won't grow or won't hatch in a cycle.

14th October 2012:

We tested again today just in case as we had tested a day early. Sadly, it still says negative.

Yesterday we held each other all day with sadness. Today we both feel anger that this is happening. How could we have two grade one embryos put back and nothing takes?

I hate this wretched feeling of sadness. We put so much effort and money in to this dream that we are chasing. Distraught.

Things go through your mind such as 'how can so many nasty people in the world have children and we can't'? And I hate this feeling of self-pity. But once again I say, people go through far worse than us...and kind people too.

It's just such a relentless game. But then, IVF is relentless I guess.

Raef actually said something to us recently that has made sense: "IVF is the same as trying naturally in that you usually have to try several times before it will actually work." So many people assume that IVF will be a one-off quick fix solution. It's clearly not always.

29th December 2012:

Some Happy IVF News:

Two weeks before Christmas I got a call from a lady called Heidi from The Lister who asked if I could confirm that I had entered their annual draw for a free IVF cycle. We had indeed, but had not thought much about it since people apply from all over the world. I replied that we had. And I must be honest, I then expected her to say 'sorry...' But to my utter surprise and excitement she informed me that having looked at our application and history, The Lister had selected us (25 cycles were being given away by The Lister in total). Tears were streaming down my face. She started informing me what I needed to do now but my mind was just full of joy and I actually couldn't hear much or speak for the tears. I just kept thanking Heidi and asked her to pass our thanks on to all involved in this decision that meant too much for words to describe. It meant we could try again but without the financial pressure this time, while also making us feel like we finally had a touch of luck on our side. I mouthed to Paul who was sat beside me as best I could through the tears that we'd got it. He too had tears and kept repeatedly, "Say thank you to them all from me too."

After all that had happened this year, the ruptured ectopic pregnancy, the negative cycles, the miscarriages, and in addition business worries and tragically a very our dear friend of ours passing away, it felt so good to finally hear some good news. We were overjoyed and still are, and still can't quite believe it.

So, now the plan is that if they can squeeze us in for a cycle in January, we will go again. Watch this space. Fingers and toes crossed as always. Feeling positive! What a Christmas present.

It's so nice for us both to be crying happy tears for a change.

'Free' 10th IVF Cycle

8th January 2013:

The first scan was four days ago. Just the preliminary scan to check that all is OK for the next cycle.

We saw Alison, (our sonographer) who was lovely as always. All looked fine in the scan. So it's full steam ahead…again.

10th January 2013:

Second scan: Nine follicles are so far doing well. Raef Faris popped out to see me briefly in the hallway in between appointments which was kind. As always his positivity was infectious and lifted me.

It's so nice to feel that I have such a strong support network at The Lister.

The nurses all also seem genuinely thrilled that we were chosen for a free cycle.

Physically, I am feeling bloated due to the follicles growing steadily now which is normal.

11th January 2013:

Third scan: Nine follicles in total are still doing well. Apparently, I may have to come back tomorrow for another scan depending upon my blood test result (hormone level), if not in two days' time.

I have felt very emotional and tired over the last few days. I am finding it hard each time I inject as some nights, due to my Gonal F dose, I am having to do three injections in one go. I am struggling as it is in to bruises, and tearful when doing it since, as I've mentioned before, each injection is a reminder to me of what we are having to go through.

Mind you, it seems to be a generally hard time in our lives too as we have lots of family and work issues which doesn't help. Paul keeps propping me up with his positive words of wisdom. Thankfully, I am especially lucky to have such a wonderful and supportive husband. Going through all of this, you need a solid and happy relationship.

14th January 2013:

Fourth scan: I have eight large follicles that are approximately the same size, which is good, with one smaller one that may catch up by egg collection.

So, The Lister have booked me in for Wednesday at 7 a.m. We are a bit concerned about snow as it is meant to be very bad this week, but hopefully it will be OK down here in the South.

So as with the end drawing near on all cycles, tonight I do my final injections, using only the trigger injection (Ovitrelle) and Orgalutran (one of several drugs that can prevent premature ovulation during fertility treatment) as I don't need any more of the Gonal F to increase the size of the follicles. The trigger injection, Ovitrelle, is used to trigger ovulation when the follicles have reached the perfect size. Apparently, they continue to grow on their own until egg collection. It is also possible that they can grow too big to be viable so it is always best to slow down the growth now at this stage.

I feel strange about Wednesday. Almost blasé, as if I'm used to it. I must get myself mentally prepared (or maybe this more relaxed approach is better).

15th January 2013:

The night before egg collection:

My mother just called me to tell me that my younger sister is having a caesarean tomorrow morning. Exactly the same time as I'll be having my operation; isn't life odd. One sister will be experiencing a joyous moment at exactly the same time one is going through this challenge.

Another baby in the family is of course such an exciting blessing though and I shall be thinking of them throughout!

16th January 2013:

Day of egg collection:

I returned to my room an hour or so ago after egg collection. I woke up very tearful this time which is unlike me. The nurse in the recovery ward was very kind and recognised me from last time (embarrassing, but I think they all know me now, from the porter to the anaesthetist).

Had the same anaesthetist as last time that really looked after me and relaxed me.

There has been a terrible helicopter accident where it's crashed in to a crane in this morning's fog just round the corner from our hospital. We can see the smoke from our window. Everyone is watching it. It's quite surreal as we can see the action, but we also have it live on the news in our room. Tragic.

Anyway, the outcome from my egg collection today is that the surgeon retrieved eight eggs out of nine follicles which is great. It's actually the same result for this stage as the ectopic, so in a way, as that was officially a pregnancy (albeit in the wrong place), we are extra hopeful.

We've just been told by Safira that seven out of eight can be injected which is actually better than the ectopic now.

17th January 2013:

Day after egg collection:

An embryologist called to say that six out of seven have fertilised which is great. They have provisionally booked me in for two days' time on Saturday at 11:40 a.m., which is a 3-day transfer. But if we hear from them by 9 a.m. Saturday it will be Monday or Tuesday. Always on call with IVF!

So now it's just drink plenty of water (from the day of egg collection until the pregnancy test itself, you have to drink two litres of water per day to flush out the drugs and prevent ovarian hyper stimulation syndrome, while also assisting with pregnancy).

Unfortunately, we had a stressful day today as it has just been unearthed that one of our favourite and key members of staff at one of our main businesses has been stealing large amounts of cash so we had to sadly dismiss him quite suddenly. Not pleasant at all. It's been hard for us both. But then, I guess one should expect such things being in business.

On top of that, there's heavy snow everywhere so we are a bit concerned about getting to The Lister if the trains are cancelled and the roads are blocked.

FACT BOX:

Ovarian Hyperstimulation Syndrome is a potentially life threatening complication that can occur during fertility treatment when there is an excessive response to drugs given to stimulate the ovaries. Symptoms include bloating, thirst, chest pains as well as others.

20th January 2013:

Today was set for the day of transfer. However, early this morning we got a call from The Lister to say that as six embryos are still doing really well we can let them go to blastocyst stage, which is booked for Monday (the blastocyst stage occurs when there are a good group of embryos and so there are no clear leaders. In other words, the results are looking excellent). We are so happy as this is excellent news and shows that they are great quality too.

Five are grade one! What a relief, but at the same time we are cautious as not to upset our emotions again.

I keep thinking how strange it is that my body has improved fertility-wise with time. This shouldn't be possible. When you look back at the beginning of our journey, our results seem to be getting better. But as always with IVF it is still a gambling game for anyone entering it. For us, we now feel so knowledgeable on this subject; I'm sure we could take a degree in it!

We have just had what has become the heaviest snow in years over night so we are still slightly anxious about how we will be getting to London tomorrow – if the trains are cancelled we will have to try to drive. It's not an option to not go.

21st January 2013 (Morning):

Due to the snow, we left our house to drive up to London an hour early (6 a.m.). En route, I received a call from an embryologist at The Lister to say that three embryos are still doing well. However, as they have not quite reached the blastocyst stage yet they would like us to delay the transfer to tomorrow morning or this afternoon. So, mid-way on the motorway, we had to change direction and return home. I'm very nervous indeed now! But this is good news really, I think. We still have to expect that they may not make it to blastocyst at all, but this would mean that they wouldn't have done so inside me anyway. You have to be quite pragmatic about it. If they are viable, they would take inside me. If they are not viable, they would not take in the laboratory under the microscope.

However, they may just be slow at turning.

As we are both so worried, I called Raef for his advice (he's been great at keeping in touch with us texting, calling and emailing us back). He said that often embryos can just be 'slow' and not to worry, and that this could be a good sign.

21st January 2013 (Afternoon):

I just had a call from an embryologist to say that this afternoon two of the embryos are looking as though they are progressing in to lovely blastocysts. Our hearts are still pounding. But all we can do now is wait until tomorrow morning.

If they don't call us, it is good news and we can have them put back in at our morning appointment. If they call us, it'll be because the two didn't make it...embryos can simply arrest and give up for no known reason.

I fear a sleepless night worrying is upon us.

22nd January 2013 (Morning):

We are now on the train on our way to London, as thankfully we didn't get 'the call'. Naturally, we are still very nervous and anxious about what news we will have when we get there.

What will be, will be, though. (And the trains are all running normally thank goodness).

22nd January 2013 (Afternoon):

Embryo transfer:

So the results are that one is a new emerging blastocyst and one is a morula turning in to a blastocyst. A morula is an early stage embryo consisting of cells (called blastomeres) in a solid ball contained within the zona pellucida. This is the stage before a successful embryo turns in to a blastocyst.

Dr Zahra Sougi and the nice Spanish nurse and embryologist were all so kind and kept saying that they 'don't want to see us again...only in nine months'! They're all so sweet. We also passed our friendly sonographer Alison in the corridor who told us that a lady with a similar case to ours (just as long) gave birth to twin girls today. Such stories give us such hope and really help.

It's been a strange day. When we left The Lister, we caught a black cab to take us to the station. I can only say that the driver was possibly an angel. We didn't wave him down outside of the hospital as we had walked up the road (so he didn't know where we had come from), but as soon as we got in to his cab this older man with white hair asked me if I'd been 'rubber stamped today and given the OK'? I just politely said, "I hope so."

He then said, "Hang in there love, it's all going to work out just fine for you...and I know it will!" He made such an impression on us both; we were quite stunned.

So all we can do now is wait until next Wednesday (test day – it's nearer as this was a longer transfer. It's always two weeks from the date of egg collection). With regards to the grades, we are a bit confused as at first we thought they said one is an eight A quality but then later they said a '2//'. I must ask what the '//' means.

24th January 2013:

Safira, the head embryologist who has spent so much time looking after us, educating us both on IVF, called this morning to say that she was sorry she couldn't be at the actual transfer yesterday. How sweet of her is that. We've got to know them all so well now. She talked me through in detail what the results meant.

Basically, for the embryo that was turning in to a blastocyst grade 2//, the 2 signifies the development (five being best) and the // means that the fluid and cavity were not yet at the stage to be graded with a letter.

She surprised me by informing me that even morulas on day six have a 40–50% rate of becoming a pregnancy. Which does actually make sense when you think about it, as morulas are what blastocysts are in the first place before they mature.

I informed her that I'm suffering currently with a bad cold and I worry it could lower our chances, but she said it wouldn't have any significant effect on anything. Phew!

I'm suddenly feeling disheartened this time round. Perhaps it is just that I now try to mentally prepare myself for the worst. And also I'm not feeling well. Paul is in Wales for the night for work so I called him to talk through the conversation with Safira.

Feeling sad, even though I feel we have all the support of The Lister team.

However, I have felt as though this cycle I've had to actually try to justify to some people why we are still doing this, which hurts. We wish more than anyone that we didn't have to go through this heartache, but there's no point in even explaining that.

I sometimes wonder if some people actually realise the pain of not being able to give my husband the greatest gift of all…all we dream about is our child together, a young sibling for Niomi that we may receive one day.

Meanwhile, we visited my new gorgeous little nephew (the one that was born the day of our procedure). He's such a tiny little gorgeous baby. I felt emotional for Paul when my sister said he hadn't yet held him and before we knew it the little one was put in his arms. It's difficult for anyone to understand this feeling unless you're going through it. But I proudly looked on at Paul with him in his arms and we just gave each other that knowing smile and wink that we always do. It's hard.

27th January 2013:

I'm now five days past a six-day transfer (or 5dp6dt as it is written in the lingo on fertility blogs online) and the waiting is killing me this time more than ever. I have also been convinced this entire time it hasn't worked. But I guess that's me protecting myself but secretly hoping I will be proved wrong.

Every twinge that I feel terrifies me that it's my period arriving (or AF on fertility blogs). Today I've had a few twinges. They're in my left side, same as my last two terribly painful periods which has worried me…I have been on Google of course reading other ladies'/couples' experiences (as we infertility couples do lots)… I guess just like all of them, I am simply hunting for positive stories with the same symptoms. I have had a slight dull headache for two days too but that can also be the medication.

Nobody really knows that we are going through this cycle this time. My brother, Jai, in a sympathetic way said to me the other day, "Why have you told everyone you're going through all this fertility stuff? It puts more pressure on you both." However, I had to explain to him that we haven't been telling people. We've kept all of this as quiet as is possible to do. But having experienced the ruptured ectopic, people do now know a little of what we are going through. In addition, we both now feel that with 1 in 6 couples experiencing fertility issues across the world, we should try to smash down the glass wall of taboo that surrounds infertility.

29th January 2013:

Update: 7dp6dt (seven days past a six-day transfer):

Well, tomorrow is the big test day. However, after toying it around in our minds, taking in to consideration that we have two slow growers on board, and in addition that the nurse informed us that they now advise people do the test on test day followed by another one a few days later whatever the result, Paul and I have decided to wait one more day.

It seems crazy in some ways as the suspense of not knowing is killing us. However, as Paul says, one day won't change the result. Also, when we tested in Spain with the miscarriage, it was a day late as we didn't want to risk spoiling our holiday so we waited. And then with the ectopic, we tested on the correct day, and it was negative. Therefore, I can't help but feel we seem to produce late developers.

I read in the newspaper today about hypnotherapy helping a lady. Perhaps I should try that next if there's no joy this time. And my mum texted me from Florida that in the USA they've discovered that spinach helps all areas of fertility for women. Fortunately, we eat a lot of it but I will up the intake too with the only risk of turning in to Popeye!

I've no symptoms at all right now. Everything today just feels normal. Although, I did suffer cold sweats last night and vivid dreams. And I'm very tired, but that could all be the drugs.

30th January 2013:

Update: 8dp6dt (eight days past a six-day transfer):

So, it being the day we should have tested we both woke up feeling anxious.

As we have our new kitchen being fitted imminently, we started clearing the old one which did, for a while, take my mind off things.

However, I then noticed on passing water that I had slight brown discharge, sorry for too much information, but this is a physical thing (and I know useful for couples going through this stage to read).

It was a minuscule amount. But was there all the same. I'm now terrified this is my dreaded period.

Then of course, I kept visiting the bathroom, but nothing. I've been Googling like a lunatic again in between! The conclusion? It could either be my period or 'implant bleeding' (this is when an embryo embeds and can sometimes cause some slight bleeding).

Something that concerns me though, is that my tummy is also making rumbling noises like it does with a period. Although I also had that with the miscarriage and the ectopic.

I've just been to the bathroom again and there is a little more again…tummy feeling odd.

31st January 2013:

Needless to say, I didn't sleep well. And when I did, I had nightmares. Paul went downstairs to make some tea for us at 7 a.m. so without telling him (to change our usual pattern) I quickly ran to the bathroom to test.

It was negative. Distraught. It was horrible telling Paul.

We are both lying in bed very sad now questioning how our futures may be and what we should do now. Our discussion also went along the lines of that we both feel so selfish having our house that we love so much, but for just us and Niomi (in between university) living in it. Should we move?

So, what do we do now? I personally keep thinking that we should request a biopsy on the embryos or/my lining or such.

I feel quite numb. I prepared myself in the night for it to be a negative after yesterday's symptoms…but I still feel very numb (I can tell that Paul does too).

1st February 2013:

My period arrived in full flow in the end yesterday. Since the ectopic episode, I now seem to feel on edge that I could have another one, as with that episode I initially had a negative test followed by what I thought was my period…paranoid I know.

Then last night we had some very important meetings at our business interviewing a new General Manager…we interviewed seven candidates, one after another. It's such an important role as whoever fills it will be our right hand person at that business, so it was difficult keeping focused at such important meetings. I felt incredibly tired with a headache throughout. This was followed in the early hours of this morning by waking up with an almighty migraine which made me sick all night. I'm in bed now and still feeling bad, but have taken Co-dydramol that I was given with the ectopic (but never used) as my head was excruciating. Yes, I gave in to painkillers. I'm feeling rubbish still. And so upset.

We both keep saying that something must be going wrong for the embryo's to not have implanted again. Why do they keep arresting or not implanting? Maybe some test will be invented in 20 years' time that could diagnose it easily. Who knows?

6ᵗʰ February 2013:

One of the parts we always dread after a failed cycle is calling the hospital to let them know.

So this time I plucked up the courage to email Raef Faris yesterday instead. I also cc'd Mr Dooley to keep him in the loop. And I requested if possible for Safira (embryologist) to attend our next meeting with him. There is always a re-group meeting after a failed cycle.

Mr Faris emailed me back to say Safira will call me to arrange a meeting date and how sorry he was. Mr Dooley also emailed back saying to call him after I've met with them, and how sorry he was.

Safira then called me. We booked the meeting. She also said that every Tuesday they hold a big group meeting with all the consultants. In the one next week she said she's going to take my (huge) file with her and ask everyone to look at it in great detail and see if there is anything being missed. I really appreciated this.

In the meantime, I've been Googling a lot this time for answers or any new IVF news.

So, any notes I have I will be taking to our next meeting, while also asking how their group meeting went discussing our case. I am also planning to ask about the PGS test (it's a pre-implantation genetic screening test on the embryo) that I've read about.

I'm really hoping something arises.

Looking on the internet, you must always be careful in this infertility game. As with illnesses that have no cure, there are a lot of sharks out there claiming that they can help you…for a lot of money usually.

In my opinion, it is wise to only speak with the truly reputable professionals. You can also ask your fertility clinic their advice on anything you may find. For example, Paul and I came across the miracles of taking daily doses of DHEA (dehydroepiandrosterone) capsules. We read that it was a huge 'breakthrough' in the infertility world to 'increase the woman's ovarian reserve'. Naturally, we jumped at the chance and paid over £100 for some to be delivered from USA. We then discussed it with Dr Michael Dooley who informed us that there are very good, and concerning, reasons that DHEA has not been legalised to be used in conventional fertility treatments in the UK, or sold over the counter here. From there not being any evidence or trials yet done on DHEA in the UK to the fact that there are some terrible and risky side effects (for example permanent hair loss), we decided to not use it. It's still in our kitchen cupboard!

And so, that was another wasted investment in something we just happened to read was a 'miracle'. You have to be so careful. From now on, any other miracle treatments that we read about will be run past our team of specialists beforehand!

There are so many people and businesses on the internet saying they have the 'answer to infertility, just pay'. However, infertility is usually a physiological and individual problem, so think about it, how can they really help through the internet more than a hands-on professional doctor? But when you're desperate you'll do almost anything…and they know that.

If, however, you find something does help you to relax at this quite traumatic time, for example fertility massage or acupuncture, then that's another matter; anything that helps you relax, do it.

22nd February 2013:

I have been extremely low today which took me by surprise. There's been lots on the news about the cut-off age for NHS IVF cycles being put up to 42 for women, so maybe that's triggered it. I am now 38.

It still seems so unfair to me that couples like us, where one partner already has a child, are not even entitled to a single NHS IVF cycle. Why are people like me (single parents) treated as if we have committed such a terrible crime (no consideration is even given to how they became a single parent). And mostly, how terribly unfair is that to Paul? The person who does not even have a child.

On top of that, we've visited a lot of new babies lately. When you are going through infertility, it doesn't upset you in the way that 'it's not your baby' when you see them, it just reminds you in a very clear way of what you can't have together. We both adore babies and children too. It's a difficult emotion to deal with.

27ᵗʰ February 2013:

Notes for The Lister meeting:
Is failure due to slow growing embryos?
Why are they slow?
Can they be slow one month then normal the next?
Any genetic tests we should have?
Read on Internet about new embryo screening that increases pregnancy rates – does he know about this? It's called EEVA.
Post Meeting:
Our meeting with Raef went well; well, as well as can be expected. He answered all of our questions that we both had clearly and informatively. But most of all, he reminded us that he often sits in his chair sadly advising couples that enough is enough, and that he suggests they now stop. He strongly advised us once again that we should continue if we can. To hear that, from this man that we trust, is enough. We have been through so much and wouldn't believe a lot of doctors that we have met through this journey, but Raef we do.

With regards to his meeting with The Lister Fertility team looking at our file, he said he gained a few suggestions that they all agreed we should try. One was to try a 'scratching' of the uterus area prior to an IVF cycle. It is called Endometrial Scratching, and it does just as it says. Grim, yes but it sounds like an option to help us. The other was to try some injections called Gestone during the next cycle. Apparently, they can help to prevent miscarriage.

We concluded that these are definitely points that Raef and both of us will consider for the future. It's good to hear some positive new directions. The meeting with the team of medics brain-storming over our case has obviously helped.

11th IVF Cycle
28th March 2013:

First scan:

So, day three of my monthly cycle is here and I've been up to London again to what has become our second home, The Lister Hospital in Chelsea, to have the first scan of this new cycle. Yes…we are trying again.

This month was a very sad one for us (not only did we lose yet another close family friend – we've been to far too many funerals in the last 12 months) but on the fertility side of things, I was late with my cycle this month. Albeit five days, but for my body clock that's a lot. So we did get quietly excited that 'maybe' our dream had finally happened naturally after all this time. All of the professionals have always reminded us that it could still happen naturally after all.

But no, hey ho, here we go again.

I'm personally feeling very nervous at the moment and if I'm honest, a bit negative this time. So I'm very aware I need to change my mindset ASAP.

When we were at the hospital today, we did laugh though, because virtually every member of the staff at The Lister came over to have a friendly chat with us in the waiting area, like old friends. One of the nurses said, "It's lovely to see you both back again. How are you both?" We do both feel a bit embarrassed, which I know is silly. I swear that even the hospital cleaner gave us a familiar glance and smile today! But as we always do, Paul and I sit in the waiting area trying to keep our spirits up so we did chuckle about this.

So tonight, I start the injections in to my tummy…here we go again jumping back on that roller coaster!

1st April 2013:

Second scan:

The results so far are as follows: The right side is showing 4–7 follicles coming through, while the left side is showing 5–6. This is looking good. Yes, I am getting more positive about this cycle!

We've been invited to a couple of friends' parties and dinner parties lately, but as I've had a really bad cold we've had to decline. It's very difficult, because since the ectopic episode everyone pretty much knows now what we are going through, albeit they don't know for how long or the exact details. And the trouble with it being public knowledge is that every time we decline an invitation either because we're already busy or like now for example me being unwell, I know that some people are assuming it's because we cannot face seeing them. I have found this especially with some people with children or babies. For example, last week when I mentioned to a friend that I was sorry we could not attend their BBQ as we were already booked to be elsewhere, her retort to me was, "Verity, I understand how hard it must be for you being around babies so please don't explain." While this, yes, could make me cross, I've also learnt through this experience, and through life's experiences, that I just have to bite my lip and let people assume whatever they want to about us. I would just look and feel even more stupid trying to convince them by saying, "No, we really are fine actually around other people's babies. We genuinely are busy that night!" I know people mean well too. So we just have to let it go.

2nd April 2013:

I was called by The Lister last night to come in early today as my routine blood test from yesterday showed that my oestrogen levels were fairly high. I've never had this before.

Fortunately, having now been up to the clinic, the scan today has shown that the larger follicles have slowed down a bit and the smaller ones have increased in size. The long and short of it all is that the hospital are not worried which is good.

We sadly have our friend's funeral on Friday (so I cannot attend the hospital that day). They would therefore like me to go in tomorrow and then again on Saturday. Raef Faris really is keeping a close eye on me which is great.

Egg collection may well then be in five days, already.

So to summarise, today's scan showed that (including the smaller follicles) I have 11–12. Nine of those are within a good size range. My lining is apparently perfect too. Once again, I find it so odd (in a good way) that my results are improving, as I am getting older. It's a mystery.

Our fingers are crossed as always!

I took a walk around our local park with my mother when I got home from London. She likes to know what's happening, and I try to be careful as I know that not only is it emotional baggage that I could potentially land on her, but also I am so knowledgeable about this whole IVF and infertility world now that I do run the risk of sounding like a fertility text book, so it's hard for people to fathom as well. I also explained to my father when he visited this week, albeit briefly, what we are going through while also explaining that 'I am fine'. We took a walk in the garden and I just gave him a brief overview of what IVF entails.

I appreciate so much that it is difficult for people not going through this directly to understand it all.

I remember a few months ago when I met a dear friend of mine who works in a superior position at Buckingham Palace. We met there, and she asked me how 'everything' was (you know when people mean the fertility subject by the frown or nod that they give you when they ask). I assured her I was fine but that it's a tough period for us. She then asked quite blatantly, (which I appreciated as no one else has) "So what exactly is IVF?"

Wow, I thought. Great, someone wants to know. I then embarked on briefly explaining what IVF involves. I could suddenly see in her face (partly gazed over and partly shocked) that perhaps I should have just summarised it and said, "It's just a few injections," which is what most people assume it is. But the trouble is, Paul and I are both so educated on the subject now, as well as respecting it as such an amazing breakthrough in our lifetimes, that it is a topic we can discuss quite freely in detail when given the opportunity. I think, though, from now on I will simplify my answer if asked again!

6ᵗʰ April 2013:

The night before last, I had a call from The Lister to say don't worry about going in that day which has saved me a journey and so I've just gone up today (Saturday morning).

The scan showed the most follicles that we have ever had! We can't quite believe it. There's 14 altogether (probably 12 that will be suitable for egg collection).

I think that the most we ever had was 11/12, so this is great news.

Therefore, I am now booked in for the op on Monday 7 a.m. So tonight at 7 p.m. I do Gonal F 375 injection as usual and Orgalutran 25 injection as usual, and then the trigger injection Ovitrelle at 9:30 p.m.

At least tomorrow night, 24 hours before the op, I get a complete break from any injections, which is always such a treat. Then it's just continuing with the tablets: Prednisolone (the steroid for my mild diagnoses of NK Cells and thyroxin, as I am borderline with high thyroid levels), and then Cyclogest twice per day after the operation (morning and night, this is progesterone to prevent miscarriage and sustain a possible pregnancy).

Here we go again, on this crazy fertility journey trying to gain a baby. I feel so nervous, but refuse to let it show.

8ᵗʰ April 2013:

Egg collection day:
Update 1:
It's 5:30 a.m. and we are on our way to The Lister for the egg collection, yes the big day is here.

Somehow we don't get used to these early morning trips to the hospital, the nerves still kick in. But I am sure we are not the only couple to feel like this! Although, amazingly I do feel calmer than usual within myself. In fact, this whole cycle I have, which is strange considering I started out feeling so negative.

Even with the injections each night, I just took them on and did them (sometimes in the past I have hesitated a few seconds). Quite a transition from the previous cycle, which I did struggle with.

Paul on the other hand, I can see is suffering this time round. Each time he's walked in to the room when I've been injecting, he's got quite upset. I guess it is what it represents. And I can tell that the run up to today he's been feeling quite anxious about it and for me. Once again, I think it must be so horrible for him seeing me taken off in the bed when I'm being put to sleep. I do feel for him. I keep reassuring him that I'm fine though.

Here we go!

Update 2:

The nurse, anaesthetist and the doctor have all been to visit me prior to the op.

The anaesthetist is going to perform some acupuncture while I am under, which I said is fine when she asked my permission. I'll try anything.

The doctor was the same one that I saw when I had the ectopic discovered (and incidentally looks like a grown up version of my teenage nephew, Phoenix, who is half-Greek).

So now, I'm off to the operating theatre.

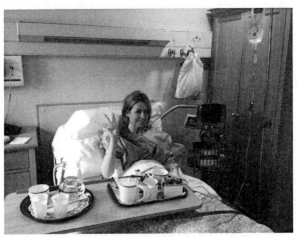

Verity after her egg collection operation

Update 3:

It went very well. It's strange but it is as if my body has started to get used to the general anaesthetic. I find that after each one, I am recovering quicker and quicker. Well, whatever it is, it's great that I am feeling much better more quickly now compared to those early days when I was taken ill.

The egg collection result was 10. Not bad. It's the second most that we've ever had, but I must admit I did hope for 11. But I shouldn't be greedy! And, I still remember those early days at the London women's clinic where they said I would only ever produce 'one black egg'.

I am home now and feel completely washed out, more than usual in fact.

Safira (head embryologist) is on holiday leave, so we haven't had a call or visit from that department as of yet to inform us of how many eggs can be injected in to. But I am sure that they will call us soon.

I spoke to a really nice senior embryologist, Katherine, the other day who told me she would oversee everything in Safira's absence but I now think possibly it was her day off too (she had very kindly told me that everyone was 'rooting for us again' as we'd been through so much, which was lovely).

But the girl today who dealt with Paul asked him if we had been before, so we are slightly anxious that we haven't received the 'extra care' that can help so much. Having said that, they are all really great here so we must have faith.

The embryologist, Katherine, has just called to see how I am and to update us.

Basically, the results so far are: eight out of 10 were injected (our magic number again). Sperm had an 88% elevated abnormality but she said this is fine as we are doing ICSI anyway. They found 52 million.

IMSI is also being done (this is when the sperm are looked at under a microscope that is 6000 times more powerful than normal ICSI microscopes. It is a recommended procedure for couples with several failed cycles behind them or a low or abnormal sperm count). Although Paul's sperm count is good, since we have had several failed attempts now, this is recommended as it increases the chances of a pregnancy anyway.

Eight grade 1 sperms were used for injecting the eight eggs. You can't get better than that.

So let's hope our little eight embryos are now tucked safely in and are doing well tonight! Katherine is calling me in the morning with an update of how they look.

9ᵗʰ April 2013:

Update 4:

OK, so Katherine called today to say that four are looking good! Phew.

Two are slower.

So all in all six are hanging in there.

Update 5:

Another embryologist has just called to say that now out of the six, one is an 8-cell grade 1, one is a 7-cell grade 1, one is a 7-cell grade 1–2, and one is a 6-cell stage 2. Two are 3 and 6 cell both grade 2. This is great news.

We go in for a morning, day five transfer on Saturday.

13ᵗʰ April 2013:

So, here we are again for the day of the embryo transfer. For some reason I've always found this one of the more nerve-wracking parts of IVF. I think it's because we get told the final quality today…and of course, it's not much fun for the woman!

Update:

The results are as follows: we had two embryos put back. It's too early to grade them now but one is an early blastocyst and one is a morula come early blastocyst.

Everyone was very positive and Paul was my rock as usual holding my hand throughout as he always has without fail.

The doctor said that with each cycle we are certainly raising our odds that it will happen one day, which I suppose is why we keep trying. All we can do now is go home and hope.

7dp5dt (seven days past a five-day transfer):

The day after tomorrow (Monday) is the dreaded test day. I can honestly say that nothing has really felt different this time, other than my nipples being slightly darker for the last couple of days which of course can be a sign of pregnancy. But I'm also aware that can also be the side effect of taking progesterone.

I keep praying and hoping. Feel like if it doesn't work now we have tried as much as we can. It's amazing how Monday morning's test result will, either way, change our lives so much.

8dp5dt:

So tomorrow is test day. We are feeling very nervous indeed. My stomach is doing knots as usual. We both keep talking about it…dreading it really. The odds are that it hasn't worked looking at our history, and I have to remind myself of this so as not to be too distraught if it's a negative again.

One horrible part of this two-week wait is that the medication you're on tricks your body in to thinking it's pregnant to prepare it if you are. How cruel is that? So basically on top of all the constant focus on every twinge you might feel wondering if it signifies pregnancy, you have to deep down also be aware that that means nothing really. Oh, this is so very hard indeed.

22nd April 2013:

Day of the pregnancy test:

Oh my goodness it says 'pregnant'!

We were both absolutely convinced it would say negative too! I had a very vivid dream last night it worked and I woke up feeling really depressed as I thought it would say negative now. Lo and behold, my dream literally came true!

I had been worrying all night. I even had night sweats.

I just spoke to Raef Faris who is also over the moon for us. He said he's been so 'emotionally involved with us', and so feels ecstatic himself. He said I'm four weeks pregnant! I simply love hearing those words! Paul and I keep saying over and over again, "We are pregnant!"

We are so (cautiously) excited. I am going to take it really easy now and hold on to this little bean!

23rd April 2013:

The day after the positive pregnancy test:

I can't believe I'm typing this…again. I feel like I'm having a déjà vu of our miscarriage in Spain. Or at least, I am worried that I am.

Yesterday afternoon, after our wonderful positive test result, I suffered some specs of bleeding. We weren't overly worried as we know that can be the so-called implant bleeding.

However, it continued on and off all afternoon. Then nothing this morning, so we were relieved.

But then, this afternoon it occurred again and became heavier. Well there's more of it and it's a deeper red, almost black. I'm now terrified, as is Paul which breaks my heart. I've had a bed-ridden day and didn't go to a staff meeting we had booked, just in case.

I am just lying here worrying now and torturing myself which is no good. Trying to think positive thoughts, but it's very hard.

Would life really be this cruel that once again when we finally get here it all goes wrong again? Please no.

I have self-prescribed myself an additional progesterone just now. I am on two per day but I have heard that more can help prevent miscarriage, so I'm upping my dose (Progesterone is the hormone given to women after an embryo transfer to prepare the lining for a pregnancy, but also to sustain a possible pregnancy).

I read a poignant saying on the Internet today: "When the world says 'give up', hope whispers 'try it one more time'…" That sums Paul and I up.

I spoke to Raef Faris. He suggested going up for a Gestone injection (a high dose of progesterone) and having a HCG blood test. But then, I suffered more bleeding the next morning so he suggested another pregnancy test…it now says negative. Utterly devastated. Bleeding lots too. Feeling shell-shocked. We are both crying lots; although, sometimes I can't even cry. I feel like we need to come to the sad conclusion that we will never have a child together…feel empty. Feel guilty too as if it is something I did. Did I get too excited by the positive test? I guess that is possible.

I read today on a medical website that when a couple suffer a miscarriage loss after IVF it's so much harder than a natural pregnancy since they've wanted it for so long, gone through pitfalls and then it finally happens but is then so cruelly taken from them. This sums up how we are feeling right now.

25th April 2013:

Miscarriage number two…

I am suffering pain now and am still heavily bleeding. This is so horrible.

I hardly cried yesterday. I just felt numb. Then last night at a family dinner at my mother's house, having put on a brave act, I escaped upstairs for a couple of minutes and cried uncontrollably alone. Cried and cried. It dawned on me that if this is the end of our journey, how terribly cruel the ectopic was. The ectopic has hit me all over again.

Also, I've been putting on an act today (our house is full of builders), which actually helps. Our house is an ongoing project that we've been doing bit by bit since we moved in a few years ago. I just escape to our bedroom now and then at the moment, especially when the pain comes on strong, like now.

It's amazing how you go through all the emotions, from feeling depressed and sad to guilty, selfish and simply empty. And then in shock at the last few days' events. This week could have been the best week of our lives as a couple.

My questions for Raef Faris when we meet for our post cycle meeting:

Gestone injections – should I have these from the day of the embryo transfer from now on? I haven't yet tried them, but have read they can assist in preventing miscarriage. Raef has always discussed them with us in the past as a possibility for us.

What can be the causes of these miscarriages I am clearly now suffering?

Are there any genetic tests that we should have done on us or the embryo?

Should I have the endometrial scratching operation now (Raef mentioned this last month to us in a meeting)?

Conclusion of our meeting with Dr Raef Faris:

Paul could have the DFI test (DNA fragmentation index), but it is expensive (thousands of pounds) and takes weeks for the results as it is sent to USA and then of course it may show nothing. And of course we are now approaching spending approx. £100,000 over these last few years on this.

Another option is for me to have a hysteroscopy with an endometrial scratching a month prior to the next cycle. It is a small operation where a laparoscopy is put inside the tummy near the belly button and some light scratching is done on the endometrial cavity. It is meant to help increase the chances of implanting in a subsequent cycle by 'scratching the lining slightly' disrupting it (which sounds horrible) making embryos more likely to settle and embed in there. At the same time, a small biopsy of the lining is taken. I've decided to have it. It doesn't sound that nice, but it may help our chances, even naturally, so I must be brave and just do it. Fortunately, I'll be having this procedure at The Lister and Raef Faris is going to do it himself for me. Apparently, it's a routine operation done everyday, so I am sure it'll be fine. Am I trying to convince myself again?

Raef, incidentally, while being sympathetic at what we had just suffered, was also very positive that we are actually getting closer to a successful pregnancy by having this miscarriage. He reminded us that it at least shows that we created a successful embryo and fell pregnant. Therefore, having now grieved, we are trying to take something positive from this horrible experience.

May 2013:

Life carries on, which does help. And we've been busy with work and various work events in the evenings lately. For instance, shortly after our last miscarriage, a close friend of ours held a business-networking event (full of some top business people in our area). As usual, we mingled and acted normal. It was held at The Grand Hotel in Brighton. Our magazine was the original media sponsor when it launched so we have always tried to attend while also supporting our friend who founded the event. As always, we met some interesting business owners from Sussex and further afield. My dear friend, the organiser, who knew what we had recently suffered, gave me a squeeze and checked I was 'OK' which meant so much in the middle of 'acting'. Like I've said before, as hard as it is to do, I believe that putting on the act does help any of us when we are suffering tough times of any sort in life.

Meanwhile, particular escapisms for Paul are his gardening (which he absolutely loves) and going to the gym. He says he can completely switch off while also being able to think and focus. I can understand that, and am also pleased he can find salvation in such things right now.

One funny thing that happened not that long ago when we were on holiday in Naples, Florida, was when an American good-looking black guy of about 25 years old came up to me on the beach when Paul was swimming and said, "Wow your husband has an amazing body for his age mam. He's probably old enough to be my dad but his body is better than mine!"

I laughed and said, "He finds going to the gym a stress reliever."

He retorted with, "Man, he must be one stressed guy!"

23ʳᵈ July 2013:

Well, today was the day I had the hysteroscopy and endometrial scratching operation. It went surprisingly smoothly. I was put to sleep and when I awoke, I didn't have as much pain as I had expected. If anyone is debating whether to have this done to increase their chances after many failed cycles, I would definitely say it's worth a try. I have also read about many successful stories from couples where the woman has fallen pregnant after this procedure.

I'm resting now, but really the after effects so far are not as bad as I had read about. Obviously, the general anaesthetic always knocks me for six and the actual operation, but while I lie here resting I feel 'OK'. Nonetheless, I am pleased it is over. It's an odd sensation though, as I feel as though I have had an IVF egg retrieval, but on the other hand I have nothing to show for it…I just go home now.

However, it's another tick in my boxes of trying anything available.

It's funny how when you're lying in a hospital bed you have time to think about things. I started thinking to myself today, 'are we being selfish? Are we putting our parents and Niomi through too much worry?' But how can we stop? It's what we long for…and I keep coming back to that point that I have this gut instinct that someday we will have a baby together. I just pray that I am right.

12th IVF Cycle

2nd August 2013:

First scan:

I am on my way to The Lister for a very early scan in preparation for the next cycle since we go away next week for our fifth wedding anniversary.

Raef Faris has allowed me to start the injections while we are away as I've been through so many cycles now I know what I am doing. I'm a bit of a 'pro' unfortunately and so we know now how my body reacts.

Further to my hysteroscopy last Tuesday, fortunately everything, as always and rather contradictorily with my body, showed up as normal. The biopsy taken flagged up as perfect. But if nothing else, we are hoping that by 'roughing' the surface as they do in this procedure and by taking the biopsy it may help an embryo embed now. Apparently, the professionals have seen this happen many times for couples in our category of 'unexplained infertility.' Although now I fear we are getting in to the 'older age' category, as time has suddenly gone by. By contrast, we were a young couple when we started this journey nearly six years ago!

It has made me think that when you hear of a woman for example who is going through IVF at 40 years plus, and you assume she started trying for a baby late, it may just be that she has been trying for say 10 years. Never judge or assume.

So here I am about to embark on possibly our final attempt cycle. Yes, that is the conclusion we are both coming to for the first time.

I must admit that I am feeling very confused lately about whether we are doing the right thing now. We both talk about it a lot and both feel the same. Should we even change our lives at this stage and start the parenting process all over? Maybe we are just trying to convince ourselves to stop, with these thoughts. Because, on the other hand, something would always be missing for us as a couple if we don't try to fulfil this dream. And we have so much love to give.

Last night, I felt very down and tearful. Most of the time, I am upbeat and smile my way through this (my mother has always said, "Fake it to make it!" It does help).

But not last night. It's probably just pre-today's appointment, feelings of going through this again.

We had Niomi's graduation last week though, which was wonderful. She graduated with a 2:1 in Law. It was the proudest moment in my life ever (other than having her of course)! In my eyes, she's simply perfect in every way, kind, intelligent, confident; I am so very blessed to have such a wonderful daughter. Should I just count my blessings and stop now? But then, what about Paul who is an amazing stepfather and longs for his own addition? And what about his wonderful mother who would make the most amazing grandmother (Paul is an only child).

Another thing that bothers us both is the wear and tear upon my body now. Although there is no evidence to prove that fertility treatments can damage the female body (as it is only encouraging the body to do something in a natural way using hormones we should already be producing), you can't help but worry.

Another concerning question that we now have is, have we wasted enough of our money? Should this 12th IVF be the last one that we dip in to our savings for? Something tells me that both of our attitudes have changed, and that if this one doesn't work, I think we will stop. In a sense, that makes us (me especially) enter in to this with a blasé attitude. I feel quite unfazed and almost laid back about it.

One thing that keeps making my mind up though when I have doubts about whether we are doing the right thing is, if I were to become pregnant naturally, (by a huge miracle now) we would be absolutely over the moon and jumping for joy to say the least! Therefore we know in our hearts that it is what we want and all the time that there is 'hope' I really do feel that we should carry on trying while we can. I guess if you were given five or six years to think about whether you really did want that dream job or car for example, it would only be natural to start having occasional doubts about whether you really did want it after all.

I have said however, that I really don't want to continue with IVF once I hit 40. It's just a personal opinion, largely since Niomi is the age she is, I do have to draw the line somewhere. Paul is in complete agreement. I see many happy women having babies in their 40s so I am all for a fit couple of any age to have babies. But like I say, I think it is because I have Niomi at the age that she is now so my situation is different.

People that know what we are going through, are so sympathetic and even say we are brave. That makes me feel guilty though in a strange way, as I don't consider us brave.

Paul and I look at this situation with typically British stiff upper lips as a card that we have been dealt in life that we have to do the best way we can with. Of course, if that means giving up one day and not sharing a child together, then of course we will. But we need to give this our best shot as once we stop, that'll be it.

We have also touched on the subject of adoption. It is something that I would like to look in to. We have always said (even before our infertility troubles) that if we have our own child one day, we would like to possibly investigate adoption. My older sister, Linda, and brother-in-law's two children are both adopted and are the most gorgeous children that have fitted in to our family as if they've always been part of it; my niece and nephew. They are the perfect little family unit. So, we have witnessed a great example of how adoption can be a happy ending for couples.

However, that is something we can only consider when and if we come to the end of this IVF road, as I think for now we have more than enough to think about and it's always so important that we focus 100% on each cycle that we embark upon.

Incidentally, my sister Linda, is one of the close people that I have been able open up to about this journey as she understands herself.

Although it is such a private experience, if there are people that care about you and who are non-judgmental, it really can help to just 'chat' over a cup of tea!

So here we go on to IVF cycle number 12 (and our 16th fertility treatment when including the IUIs)!

I've been told to inject ideally from day three of my cycle this time with Gonal F. And, I must call The Lister nurses when my monthly cycle has started while we are away.

On another note, as well as all of the other concoctions added to my diet that may help, I've been sent a newspaper article today by a close family friend about 'raspberries helping women fall pregnant'…raspberries it is then!

12th August 2013:

I had my second scan today after a wonderful few days away in Lake Como, Italy, for our anniversary. It's a truly naturally beautiful place full of serenity.

As planned, I started the injections out there as my monthly cycle began towards the end of our trip. It was a memorable break that Paul had arranged as a surprise for me; all I knew was that we were going somewhere for a week. We both fully relaxed swimming (as I can at this stage) in the Lake and enjoying the warm climate every day; the perfect way to coach my body before this forthcoming cycle!

A strange thing also happened while we were out there. Sitting on sunbeds one day at the far end of the lakeside beach, I turned and smiled at the older couple next to us who returned a smile back. Then as I lay back down on my sunbed, it hit me like a bolt of lightning who they were, or at least who *he* was. I realised that the man was none other than Professor Robert Winston (the pioneer who brought IVF to the UK and whose documentary I had watched all those years ago)!

I told Paul, who took a sneaky look and agreed it was him. We sat whispering to one another deciding whether we should say 'hello' and tell him what we were going through. But somehow we couldn't muster up the courage. And most of all, it felt rude to impose on their holiday like that. Goose pimples kept running up and down my arms. Was this a positive sign for our next cycle?

So, being terribly British, we sat a few inches away from the man who had made it possible for so many people to have children and just felt in awe. I kept saying to Paul 'fate must have sat us right next to him.' Where we were staying was a very secluded part of Lake Como called Bellagio at a hotel called Villa Serbelloni, sitting on a small ridge overlooking the water. And it wasn't even a proper beach; it was a tiny area with a single row of sunbeds and the four of us were in one little corner of it. What were the chances of us being at the same remote hotel and on sunbeds beside each other when we are at this stage in our lives?

Needless to say, not speaking to him will probably be something we will always regret. However, maybe a little of his fertility wonder will have rubbed on to us for our next cycle! Who knows?

Anyway, back to reality, today's scan has shown ten follicles are growing well with possibly some little ones coming through if we are lucky.

As I was away for a few days and the follicles are quite big now Raef wanted me to inject a larger than usual dose of Orgalutran. I actually have to take Cetrotide this time though as the pharmacy had no supply of my usual Orgalutran which has confused things for me as it is administered differently, but I am sure I will get the hang of it. Cetrotide (same type of drug as Orgalutran) has to be mixed with powder in a vial, shaken and then sucked back up the syringe using a massive needle, then carefully changed to the smaller needle to be injected (whereas Orgalutran is simply injected directly from the syringe it comes packaged in). I did use this drug once before in an earlier fertility treatment though. As today I had to have 3 mg of it (a large dose), the nurse did it for me. There was such a lot being injected in to my tummy that I was a bit shocked. But it is OK, just a sore bump now.

I am back again in three days' time for another scan.

I am starting the prednisolone (steroid tablets) tomorrow. I am staying on the same Gonal F dose as previously but no more Cetrotide now until they tell me, as the larger amount that the nurse injected will keep me going for a few days.

For some reason, it was emotional being at The Lister today, but every time I feel this I push it away again.

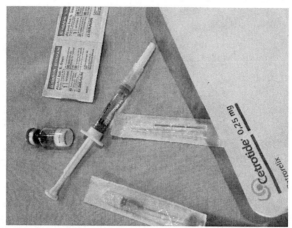

Cetrotide has to be mixed with powder in a vial, shaken and then sucked back up the syringe (pictured above)

15th August 2013:

I just had the third scan. I am now waiting for the blood test to be done and to see the nurse.

The scan showed 12 follicles are in the running now which is good. Eight are on the left side and four on the right. Some are small, but the embryologist informed us that they may let the large ones go (get too big and sacrifice them) and allow the small ones to grow through. Depending on the blood result today I may have egg collection Saturday or Monday (today is Thursday).

Have been feeling quite tearful this time. The trouble is, the more of these cycles of IVF you go through, the less everyone may comfort you as they think you're so used to it now. The reality is that it can actually be harder as time goes by. After all, we're not machines (although it feels like it sometimes).

Physically, I am feeling bloated, but no wonder with 12 follicles inside me. I am quite bruised too from the injections and very tired from the drugs, but also the steroid prednisolone keeps you awake at night.

I have just seen the nurse and had the bloods taken. They want to see me tomorrow to see how the follicles are growing so I have an appointment, unless they call to say the blood result is

OK. Also, Raef Faris would like me to start the Gestone injections in this cycle from now on. They are basically a very strong dose of progesterone that assists with pregnancy and sustaining it. They are injected directly in to the buttock muscle to get straight in to the blood stream. The plan is that the nurse will show Paul how to do it tomorrow, as unless you're a contortionist you cannot inject this one yourself. He will then do this from the day after egg collection for up to six weeks if we receive a positive test result after the two-week wait. It is meant to be very painful so I'm dreading it, but at the same time it is meant to help prevent miscarriage. So it's worth it. Paul says he isn't too happy about going back to the hospital again tomorrow. Personally, I think he is understandably worried about these injections poor thing. I must admit, I would struggle with giving them to the person I love.

17ᵗʰ August 2013:

This was the fourth and final scan of this cycle as we have been booked in for egg collection Monday (today is Saturday).

Everything is looking good and the follicles are growing well. About nine are good sized ones.

Paul had his lesson on how to inject the nasty Gestone in to me. It is actually quite complicated as we have to mix ampules and it's a very large needle (which surprised us both) that has to go directly in to my buttock muscle. The nurse teaching us admitted that it is a very painful injection (she informed us that she had to have them herself for her pregnancy). She explained that it can only go in to two areas of the buttock in order to avoid veins, so the positioning is very important – more pressure for poor Paul! Also, when Paul administers it he initially has to withdraw it slightly while it's inside me to check there's no blood withdrawing. If this were to happen, it would indicate that he's hit a vein.

This new addition is quite unpleasant and nerve-wracking. And I feel so sorry for Paul having to do it. Apparently, I will become quite bruised and so these large injections will have to eventually go directly in to bruises. Ouch.

I have to have these for two weeks (and like I say, if the pregnancy test is positive, we continue with them for six weeks further).

I really hope all this is worth it!

19ᵗʰ August 2013:

Egg collection:
Egg collection went well today.

The anaesthetist was the lady who administered acupuncture on me last time while I was under and the surgeon was Dr Zahra Sougi again. They managed to retrieve seven eggs out of the eight follicles, and we were told just before we left that seven out of the seven were mature which were great odds. So basically, seven can be injected with sperm. Now we just have to wait for the phone call tomorrow to see how they're doing.

I'm feeling OK, just a few tummy aches and extreme tiredness, but that's all normal.

20ᵗʰ August 2013:

So this morning has been a bit fraught…due to me being such a baby. Basically, today was the first morning of the horrible Gestone injections (a reminder, I am having to have these since we have suffered two miscarriages).

The injections have to be mixed from two vials using a large needle before being transferred to the medium needle that Paul has to inject into my buttock muscle. The fear of it hitting a vein has made me react like a baby! It's also not nice to have this the day after egg collection when you're feeling fatigued. So poor Paul, every time he was all set with the needle, I kept running off and saying 'I can't do this.' It was funny, but I also really didn't know if I could do it.

I eventually managed to somehow give in and let Paul do it. I had to then keep very still on my front on our bed while he slowly injected it. I do feel for him!

After all my fuss though, it really wasn't *that* bad. I now dread the part when I will be bruised and injected in to.

Anyway, the embryologist has just called me. The good news is that out of the seven injected, five embryos are doing well. Therefore we are provisionally booked for a three or six day (blastocyst) transfer. They are calling me again tomorrow with another update.

21st August 2013:

The embryologist called me to say that, now being two days later, four embryos are in the 4-cell stage at 'top quality'. This is great news. One embryo is a three cell at an average stage 2–3. Not bad.

They'll call me tomorrow before 9 a.m. if my appointment is cancelled due to the transfer being moved to Saturday hopefully! (Which would mean it's a blastocyst transfer)

Meanwhile, the Gestone injections aren't getting any easier…and yes, I am now bruised. Paul is great at handling it though. I now just clench my fists and 'try' think of other things.

22nd August 2013:

The embryologist called at 9 a.m. today to say that we still have five embryos with three doing very well and so we are to go in on Saturday (a five-day transfer). One is a seven-cell grade one. Two are eight cell, one a grade one and one is 'compacting' (this basically means that the cells are melting together in preparation for the blastocyst stage). All in all, this is a great result.

The fourth one is a seven cell, and the fifth one is a four cell, and both are of average quality. My guess is that these two are slowing down now.

But the remaining are looking promising so we are both cautiously excited (perhaps *relieved* is a better description)!

Meanwhile, even the Gestone injections are keeping me awake now; I've been dreaming about them. And it's quite horrible how bruised I am from them and how much it now hurts. I can even feel the little lumps where each injection has been, like small golf balls. I have bought some arnica cream to see if that helps alleviate the bruising.

24th August 2013:

Day of the embryo transfer:

Well, today went really well. In fact, our best results so far, which is amazing.

Results and grading of the embryos today were:

Two blastocysts were put back. One blastocyst was at the 'hatching stage' grade b2c (B=quality, 2=size, C=shell quality), while the other one was an early blastocyst but it's too early to grade that one.

There were two morulas of average grade, so we are leaving them for an extra day to see if they are fit for freezing. There are however, lower chances once embryos have been frozen (something not many people realise when investing in this procedure, financially and emotionally, as a backup for a later date).

One morula was below average, not viable.

The team was so kind as always today making jokes and chatting about every day events, but also extremely excited by our current results which boosted our confidence a lot. The embryologist, Katherine, said that the hatching blastocyst had developed so much from 7 a.m. today till our appointment at 10 a.m. that it was one of the best transfers she had ever seen! This is just amazing to hear. We are so used to receiving the bad news or being Mr and Mrs Average; to be top of the class, feels great!

In addition, and very excitingly, the hatching blastocyst 'breathed'! Yes, it actually breathed. Apparently, this is a phenomenon in IVF where the blastocyst expands and contracts. Occasionally, while the doctor is scanning you when they are about to put the embryos back in to you, this can sometimes be seen (but rarely). While the embryo was placed under the microscope and shown to us on the scanning monitor screen beforehand, Paul was fortunate enough to actually see this happen! I think that at that split second, I was looking at the other blastocyst next to it so sadly I missed it. The nurse, Sonia, also witnessed it and said it was the first time she had seen this happen (she has done hundreds of transfers apparently). She said previously she's only heard about it and was clearly excited to witness this for the first time. The embryologist, Katherine, also witnessed it; she drew our attention to it when it occurred. They all said this is a really great sign! I am now so excited and feeling really upbeat about this transfer and the results.

So, all in all we are on our way home feeling cautiously excited and elated. Come on little ones inside me! Hang on in there and grow.

25th August 2013:

I received a call today (the day after the transfer) from Katherine to say that, just as we had expected, the two slower ones were not viable for freezing, as they had slowed down a lot in the last 24 hours. Never mind though, let's just hope one of these little blastocysts that I have on board does well!

Re the nasty Gestone injections, I've discovered that creating a calm environment helps us both. I now put on some relaxing music, lay pillows on the bed for me to rest my tummy on and sprinkle lavender oil over them for me to inhale. Then throughout the day I massage arnica cream on to my bruised butt (although I don't do the area that's just been injected for a few hours so it can heal). I can't really say whether they're getting easier or not. One day it'll hurt so much I want to scream, while other days I feel hardly anything. Hence my apprehension before I have each one. And poor Paul, he is struggling with them as he feels he's hurting me. And the mixing of them, changing needles and cracking open the vials is hard for him (one vial even cut his finger). Then on top of that, he has to be sure he's injecting muscle and not a vein or a sciatica nerve (or even broken glass which is a particular fear of Paul's as occasionally small shards of glass do fall inside the vials). Oh, the joys!

28th August 2013:

4dp5dt (four days past a five-day transfer):

Paul and I have been taking it easy – thank goodness, we can work our own hours and from home. It is a luxury in this situation.

The weather has been gorgeous so today we went to the beach for a sneaky couple of hours and enjoyed ice creams. It was very relaxing! Paul had a swim but as I can't I just went up to my knees (it is not recommended to swim or have a bath once the embryos have been placed back).

I have had some stomach cramps today though, so naturally I keep worrying which doesn't help me... I am so anxious. These two-week waits don't get any easier.

30th August 2013:

6dp5dt:

Have felt incredibly tired today. I even struggled to get dressed and out of bed. I think the drugs have all well and truly kicked in.

I have had tummy cramps for a couple of days now.

We have been out for lunch today with friends. It was a really relaxing afternoon at a local country gastro pub. We sat outside soaking up the sun. It was nice to not have to discuss our IVF (as they don't know) and just laugh and have fun. My stomach felt so bloated! Ironically, I think look a few months pregnant. Another ironic cruel trick of IVF. It could be the Cyclogest (progesterone drugs).

The bruises on my butt are now black and purple. It's like I have a golf ball sized tattoo on each cheek. Very attractive I'm sure!

I keep worrying that it hasn't worked...then I try to convince myself that it could work this time, since we have tried even harder than usual with the laparoscopy operation prior to this cycle and these new Gestone injections, and then we had our excellent blastocyst results (of which Paul saw one 'breath.') But also I am very aware that for no reason at all it might simply not work. Gosh, this is so hard. I am debating like this in my mind every day, as is Paul I know because then we do it together out loud! What fun. Tonight we are going to enjoy a light barbecue with Niomi, followed by a comedy (a glass of wine for Paul after my injections) and probably some chilled pineapple juice for me – yes, apparently pineapple juice can assist with implanting! But you have to time it carefully, as pineapple is also thought to cause miscarriage when consumed in early pregnancy by some cultures.

31st August 2013:

7dp5dt:

Well today was my lovely dad's 80th birthday (even though he looks and seems in his 60s. Really!). We held a party for him on the roof terrace at our restaurant at lunchtime and it was a super day with lots of friends and family.

The only thing was that at the end of it, I did start to worry, *have I overdone it today?* I hope not. I did stand for a long time. But then again, and as Paul reassured me, you can become paranoid about what you're doing. I think I am. Because then we got a Thai take away in the evening and I became worried about the spicy hotness of it affecting things. So much is relying on this…so I guess it's natural to worry.

I've no symptoms at all today and the cramping has been gone for a couple of days now. I am just suddenly feeling bloated this evening. But that's probably the Thai food!

Naturally I keep worrying that it hasn't worked, and when I look back at my notes for my previous cycle (albeit resulting in a miscarriage) I find myself comparing symptoms (as in early pregnancy symptoms) and I feel different this time without those symptoms. It's terrible how you end up analysing everything.

Of course though, I pray it's worked, but I'm testing the morning after tomorrow and today I feel a tad doubtful if I'm honest.

Meanwhile, Niomi has launched an online lifestyle blog today so I can now happily sit back and read about what she's been up to. This first one has already proved so popular too with hundreds of lovely comments to her from people enjoying reading it all over the world. She's a natural writer.

1st September 2013:

8dp5dt

Well, needless to say, we've both been anxious today as it's the day before test day. It's also Sunday so having nothing in the diary, it's been hard keeping myself busy! We went to a garden centre and then did the usual Sunday chores at home, and then I cooked Niomi, her boyfriend Marcus and us a roast pork dinner (again, I hope I didn't overdo it. But it was an enjoyable evening and meal). We all played scrabble afterwards which was fun. What a civilised Sunday!

The trouble is, I've had this sinking feeling that it hasn't worked. And if it is a negative, I am obviously dreading tomorrow. The thing is that when we are in this current state of waiting, we can almost 'hope' and pretend to ourselves that I am pregnant. Once we receive a negative (as we have so many times), that bubble of hope is burst and turns to despair. It's horrible not knowing how we will be feeling this time tomorrow.

Well, it's out of our hands now and so it's over to fate.

This is so hard.

2nd September 2013:

Test day:

Well, I'm still shaking as I write this, in disbelief. Wow, the test says 'pregnant'! Elated and so incredibly surprised, shocked, and so, so happy…and so many other emotions that I just can't think of right now. I'd convinced myself all night that it hadn't worked, especially as I've had no symptoms. Take note ladies currently in the two week wait with no signs!

I woke up at 6 a.m. bursting for the bathroom, and waited as long as I could as I almost didn't want to do it. Then Paul and I decided that to change our usual pattern I go downstairs to do the test. I hadn't even finished 'doing it' when it started flashing 'pregnant' at me. The timer was still flashing too. So when I handed it to Paul, we were cautious in case it changed again, as it still hadn't finished flashing. Then it stopped and said 'pregnant 1–2 weeks'! So happy!

In IVF, you add on weeks to account for the egg retrieval and transfer, so I think I'm officially just under one month.

The strange thing is that we both feel very cautious this time, rather than getting *too* excited. We don't have that ecstatic feeling we've had in the past with the miscarriages for example, and I think that's due to our previous experiences. I can only describe it as crying with happiness while also being terrified inside.

However, this time the blastocyst 'breathed', and now the test turned to pregnant early so we are hoping these are all good signs.

Hurray…so far!

3ʳᵈ September 2013:

The morning after the positive pregnancy test:

Head embryologist at The Lister, Safira, has just called me. She said she was off yesterday and just came in to work with her team excited all saying to her: "You won't believe who is pregnant!" She asked who and they told her it was me, and she said they all cheered with her in the laboratory! She said she simply had to call me as she was 'so over the moon'. How amazing is that to hear from the embryologist who has helped us so much. She and her team really have gone over and above in a way rarely seen in medicine. I explained that we are *cautiously* elated. She said that when we go to The Lister in two weeks' time for our first pregnancy scan we must pop in to see her. She is a very special person indeed.

Although this has been at times a horrific journey, one way that we have been very lucky in is that the team at The Lister have shown such care and support that I don't think we would have received anywhere else.

Anyway, physically now I do feel that everything is just different this time to the previous pregnancies. Somehow, it feels more 'normal' and 'settled', I even felt a bit queasy this morning, but I may be imagining it (or it could just be all of the excitement and shock). Paul is so elated, which is so lovely to see. Even sharing this early pregnancy together so far feels simply amazing. We have been through so many tough experiences that having this special moment together right here and now is just wonderful. We can't stop grinning!

6ᵗʰ September 2013:

Four days after the positive test:

Apart from being elated and it being on my mind every minute of every day, I've actually had no symptoms so far (if putting the above mentioned sickness down to excitement). The bruises on my buttocks are a bit painful and itchy still (like gigantic mosquito bites, but worth it) and that's all. We have to obviously continue with these injections now for six weeks.

I have been waking up early, but I think that's all the excitement. Paul and I keep planning way ahead now which I know seems crazy, for example we even discussed briefly the nursery, but we do it cautiously as we think that positive thinking must also help. I am so focused on holding on to this pregnancy if I can!

We are having our first scan in a week and a half on 19th September when I'll be six and a half weeks pregnant (I still love saying those words). Fingers crossed for it. I'm just trying to do everything slowly and keeping calm. It's so lovely seeing Paul so happy too! I can't put that in to words.

We are also in the middle of purchasing a new business. It's a Japanese AA Rosette restaurant and cocktail bar in mid-Sussex. The biggest business we've ever bought together in fact, so it's a major deal with a lot to manage. For obvious reasons, I've backed off from it and Paul is so superb so it's working just fine.

We are not sure when to tell our parents about our pregnancy. My mother and stepfather, Ian, go away for three months next month to America so we are debating whether we should tell them before they go or on Skype when they are there. We don't want people worrying about us either so it might be nicer once we have hopefully been given the 'all clear' with a scan.

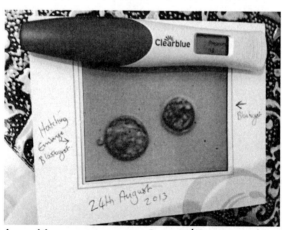

Verity's positive pregnancy test from 2nd September (top), with the image of the hatching embryo (left) and blastocyst that 'breathed' (right) from her embryo transfer on 24th August

10th September 2013:

5 weeks pregnant:

Here we are having made another week; a week after the pregnancy test. This is such an achievement for us. This is just amazing.

Everything feels normal too. No symptoms. Only tender breasts (but that's most likely all the progesterone I'm taking), and I am popping to the bathroom frequently (but that could be the two litres of water a day I'm consuming). I decided to carry on drinking that much water as I'm on such large doses of the Gestone injections and Cyclogest capsules, I figured it needs to be flushed out of my system.

I have turned in to the biggest worrier on this earth, but I have since read that that is normal with IVF pregnancies and I guess looking at our history of now having had twelve IVFs, miscarriages and the ruptured ectopic pregnancy, and all the failures along the way that's understandable. Our first scan is next week, so I'm hoping that if it is all OK (fingers crossed it will be) I may feel more reassured and start to relax a bit. So much is relying on this forthcoming scan.

We went for a short country walk yesterday which was really nice and then we had a dear friend's 30th birthday in the afternoon. I'm finding it so hard not telling people our news; we both are. We want to shout it from the rooftops and tell the world!

We've decided that we both want to tell Niomi first, then hopefully after the scan have Paul's mother and stepfather, John, with my mother and stepfather, Ian, for dinner and tell them all then, followed by my father and his partner, Janet…and then after three months, the masses I guess!

We are so excited to tell all of our parents. For Paul's mother, this will be her first grandchild. I know it will be a very emotional time telling her as she has felt the often-distressing times of this journey with us; she has seen our tears.

We keep randomly saying to each other each day 'we are pregnant'! We can't quite believe it! We are so very happy…but still cautiously so. It's a strange feeling as nothing feels different at the moment so it's easy to forget…then we have to pinch ourselves that this *is* actually happening. Every day is a milestone for us. And, we are just ecstatic to reach those milestones. Every morning we keep saying, "Another day and I'm pregnant!" Please God, look after this little bean this time for us.

12th September 2013:

5 weeks and 3 days:

As I've still had no symptoms I decided to do a sneaky pregnancy test to check that everything is still OK. And fortunately, it came back positive again but had also increased in weeks (the first one said 1–2 weeks, this one said 2–3 weeks. Although, as I mentioned earlier, in IVF you add on weeks so I'm actually officially just over five weeks). This is a great feeling and a huge relief!

I feel so happy. It all seems just 'right' this time too, as though everything has finally clicked. Although, I am of course so anxious for the scan a week today. Just praying that everything will be OK.

Paul and I had a coffee with my mother yesterday and then a few minutes afterwards we bumped in to her in the street and she asked, "Is everything OK…health wise? I've just been thinking…"

We were so surprised by her asking this…we both very vaguely answered her, "Yes, fine thank you." We felt (and probably looked like) guilty teenagers.

She shocked us even more by then asking outright, "Are you pregnant?"

We couldn't believe it! I just mumbled, "We are in the waiting game and just don't want to talk about it but we are really fine thank you." The 'waiting game' was the expression I always used to her to describe the two week wait. Little did she know that the dinner at our house I'd booked in our diaries for next week was actually when we planned tell her after the scan.

She said, "Well if you are pregnant, you should be resting." Mother's intuition!

As we are in the middle of buying a new business, I think she's worried I'm over doing it if there is a possibility of me being/falling pregnant.

And of course, I am pregnant! But I'm resting whenever I can and trying not to get stressed about anything. I actually feel great. Happy!

17th September 2013:

5 weeks and 6 days pregnant:

Starting to feel slightly worried, as I don't have any symptoms. I have these fears in the back of my mind that it's stopped growing or something; past experience has taught me that this can happen. Out of nowhere today I've had this feeling of doom. The scan isn't until four days' time. It seems like forever waiting for it. Maybe it's just the anxiety of waiting affecting me.

We went for dinner to our new Japanese restaurant last night and I just felt so washed out by 9 p.m. (probably due to the injections, plus our little cat phoebe has been keeping us awake every night so I've been awake from 5 a.m.)!

I think Paul finds it hard that I feel worried, tired and just want to be at home curled up on sofa at the moment. But after these last few years of ups and then downs, I just feel like I could have a time bomb inside me some of the time and need to rest just in case. The trouble is, our social life has gone in to full swing with so many invitations…it's typical. And understandably, Paul wants us to go to things. And why shouldn't we? I'm just being overcautious, I know. For example, he wants us to get a train across Europe in a couple of months to our friend's party that we've been invited to in Spain (rather than fly). It would be an amazing experience and I'd so love to go to their party! As much as I really, really want to go (it would be so lovely), the idea of travelling in a train for that long away from our hospital fills me with dread. Is it really wise to go? My heart says we shouldn't. So I'm not sure what we will do.

We also have another friend's birthday party this weekend, which will be a late night one. I'm wondering if rather than leaving early if I should miss it altogether. But then, it'll look odd Paul going alone. Oh…the predicaments. I wish I could just be wrapped up in cotton wool to be honest.

In addition, I feel like I've convinced myself it's stopped growing now which is just horrible. I'm also sure I'm not visiting the bathroom as often as I was. You start to analyse everything which is testing.

I need to see how the scan results are and go from there.

17ᵗʰ September 2013:

6 weeks 2 days:

I'm feeling slightly more positive now. I've been stalking IVF and pregnancy forums on the Internet, and read about a lady who said she's been suffering exactly the same as me – she was going to the bathroom a lot and now nothing and she's at the same stage as me. She went for her 6-week scan, and all was fine! And the doctor told her it is normal for symptoms to come and go. Let's hope. I am very, very tired again and am waking earlier every morning – 6 a.m. today. And I'm already a self-confessed non-morning person!

19ᵗʰ September 2013:

We are both feeling very nervous this morning; to be expected though as it's the day of our six-week scan.

I've also woken up with a headache, the only one of this pregnancy so far. It might just be the worry.

One second we are both excited planning how, all going well, we will tell my parents at dinner tomorrow night and then Paul's parents when they are back from their holiday (yes we made a change of plan of telling them all together when we realised Paul's parents were away). Then the next second we panic and almost prepare ourselves for things to go wrong, as we know only too well they can.

It's now 8:20 a.m. and the scan is at 12:45. Here we go!

19ᵗʰ September 2013:

The 6-week scan:

We both feel totally overwhelmed; we saw the little heartbeat beating away! Tears all around…including many from The Lister team that has looked after us all this time.

Dr Raef Faris was waiting outside of the scan room nervously pacing the corridor like an expectant father when we came out. We gave him the thumbs up and we all hugged and shed tears. Then Dr Marie Wren, who put the most recent embryos back inside me, came to see us and was also overjoyed. Liz, our sonographer, scanning this time, was the same. We requested to see Safira as she had asked me to, and again she too was overjoyed and had tears in her eyes. It's been an overwhelming day and also very surreal. So often, we've been at The Lister feeling down in the dumps. This feeling is simply amazing; I wish I could bottle it.

We are of course still cautious. Dr Marie Wren suggested we ask who the best obstetrician in our hometown is and also request a ten week scan as opposed to waiting for a twelve week one. And to inform our GP that due to our history and journey, the doctors at The Lister have advised we come under the 'special pregnancy care' bracket.

I am so pleased that we have reached another massive milestone today!

I am just bursting to tell the world right now.

20ᵗʰ September 2013:

The day after the six week scan:
Today, I am 6 weeks plus 6 days pregnant.

The night of the scan, we sat down and told Niomi the happy news, which was so wonderful. Another huge significant moment. She is overjoyed. But like us is of course cautious as well telling us that we shouldn't get too excited just in case. It's so sad in many ways how this experience has affected all of us.

Then last night I cooked dinner for my mother and stepfather and we told them. There were happy tears all around! And again, lots of discussions of caution.

However, during dinner I went to the bathroom and to my absolute horror I saw some light red blood. I returned to the table and acted normal and carried on with the evening, somehow, without telling anyone...not even Paul. I kept visiting the toilet. It happened one more time and then nothing. I decided to take an extra Cyclogest (progesterone) as I recalled with a previous bleed (albeit which resulted in a miscarriage) that Michael Dooley advised me to take an extra one to stop the bleeding. As previously mentioned too, I also know that progesterone can prevent possible miscarriage.

When my parents had gone, I gently informed Paul. He was amazingly calm, sent me to bed and said 'what will be will be'. I know he was devastated and worried though like me.

I was awake most of the night as a result, so was Paul, but fortunately I didn't suffer any more bleeding.

However, I am now sitting downstairs at 8 a.m. and have just suffered a small amount more. I am panicking like mad. Its Saturday too so I can't do anything doctor-wise. Why do these things always happen on weekends? My tummy is also making slight grumbling noises/motions reminiscent of what you get during a period, and what I also got during the miscarriages.

I am unsure how I should feel. If I'm too upset, it could start and even encourage something nasty to happen. But also maybe I should prepare myself now mentally for the worst. I am just not sure.

I don't want to text Raef as it's the weekend and by his own admission the other day 'he is 100% emotionally involved in this pregnancy'!

I feel so scared to even move my tummy. Am just going to rest today and tomorrow.

Paul is at one of our friend's parties tonight at our restaurant. I guess I will just have a couch and pyjama evening and try not to worry. I just pray that all will be OK. How can we go from seeing a heartbeat to this in 24 hours?

Later that day:

So, we decided to text Raef after all as we were panicking so much. He called me back immediately upon reading my text and said I'm on the full dose of all the medication so not to take any more (Gestone injections and Cyclogest). He also reassured us that this can be very normal in early pregnancy and not to worry. He is not concerned. He said 90% of cases where this happens turn out to be fine. He also very kindly offered me an extra scan for next week to hopefully reassure us, which we are going to book Monday. He joked that we probably want a scanning machine at home now! I said Paul will be on eBay buying one tonight now that he's said that!

Talking to him has reassured me a lot. He sounded relaxed, which calmed me down. He also warned me that I should be aware that when I stand up or walk up and down stairs there might be more of this small bleed. Apparently, if it's implant bleeding, it's purely due to gravity and I shouldn't worry.

So we are just hoping that it is simply that.

21ˢᵗ September 2013:

6 weeks 6 days:

Thankfully, the bleed has stopped completely. It's such a relief. I've been worried sick, although Raef's reassurance and advice helped so much.

Paul was out last night and as always I'm no good at sleeping alone so I didn't then sleep till around 6 a.m. So I am feeling exhausted to say the least.

I can't believe I'm seven weeks pregnant in the morning. I've read up on the Internet about how much the baby develops in this coming week. It's quite extraordinary. I just want to skip ahead to three months, so I feel a bit more secure about it.

7 weeks 2 days:

The bleed had stopped for a few days, but then when I woke this morning I had a small amount again which concerned me/us.

In the end we decided that we weren't going to take Raef up on his offer of the extra scan but now as it has started again we've decided to and so I am booked in for tomorrow. Very nervous. I asked the nurse on the phone if we should be concerned and she said that basically it could just be 'old blood' from implantation (especially as it's a deep red). I do hope so!

Post scan:

So today at seven weeks and three days, we had our second scan and I'm so pleased and relieved to report that everything was fine. The little heartbeat was beating away fast.

We were both so nervous, again. Even Alison who scanned us this time said she was nervous too! She was the person who discovered my ectopic pregnancy last year though, and said today how she remembered it well and how cruel it was.

However, here we are now nearly touching on two months pregnant, and all is looking good.

As we left we bumped in to the kind Spanish nurse, Sonia, who has been with us each time that we have had embryo transfers. She was the one who also saw our embryo 'breathe' this time with Paul. We told her our good news today and like all of them, there she was so happy for us.

We then departed to get a taxi (after a thyroid blood test), and Raef Faris came running down the road looking worried asking, "How was it?" We quickly told him how everything is looking great and thanked him again. He's been such a big part of this journey!

So now, as crazy as our lives usually are, after we sat on some deck chairs for half an hour in Hyde Park having had a celebratory lunch in 'Nobu' (no sushi for me though)! Paul went on to a meeting regarding a new venue opening in London. Also, the new business that we are purchasing is finalising today (a Japanese fine dining restaurant, so today's lunch is also research)! Phew, what a day. Meanwhile, we have a new general manager starting at our Brighton restaurant so we are popping in there this evening.

I'm now taking a break on the sofa for a while so as to relax in between all of this. Think I'm getting the balance right.

So overjoyed by the scan…just want to jump up and down, and tell everyone!

3rd October 2013:

Feeling completely exhausted. Blood pressure is low so perhaps that's why (as well as it being the first trimester). My blood pressure today was 93/56 with 97 beats per minute.

8 weeks and 4 days pregnant:

Feeling well with still very little symptoms – only very tired, a lot of bathroom trips and bloated tummy. Nothing else.

Sadly though, our gorgeous young Siamese cat Phoebe went missing three days ago, which has been upsetting for us all. Feels like déjà vu with our previous cat, Coco, all over again. Hoping she'll turn up! But starting to lose hope now. As a late dear friend of ours, the author James Herbert, said to me the last time I saw him, "God giveth with one hand and taketh with the other…" such poignant true words. So often that happens.

I'm hoping the stress of losing our little cat has not affected me physically so I'm trying to keep calm.

Meanwhile, in the last 24 hours we've exchanged on our new business. It's very exciting, even if not ideal when I'm pregnant.

But again, I'm trying to rest and so have taken more of a back seat than usual by avoiding some of the meetings.

I am seeing our new GP today for the first time. Feels funny to be off The Lister register in a sense now, and on the 'normal' pregnancy route.

9 weeks pregnant today:

So, we met our new GP last week who was very nice and completely understood our cautiousness and worries after what we've been through to get here. She agreed that we should have a ten-week scan, and is emailing our local hospital to request it telling them of our full history. She also suggested that if by any chance they say no, we should do it privately.

Today I woke up with an unfortunate migraine and so, as always with me and migraines, was sick several times (our little cat Phoebe has never returned, so maybe it's the upset from that).

It's later now, so I am feeling much better, but very washed out and tired. Paul's been looking after me. He's been great. I'm worried that all the nutrients have gone from my body, but as Paul rightfully says morning sickness doesn't do any harm so why should this sickness. Once again, for obvious reasons, I am worrying. I still have to pinch myself each morning that I am pregnant.

Having my daily Gestone injection during a migraine was not the most pleasant experience I must say! But still, these nasty little needles could be what are helping us hold on to this precious pregnancy so it's all worth it, with or without a migraine.

I'm still so sad about our little cat, Phoebe, who never came home. She's only a cat I know, but one we love so much, so I just keep hoping she'll walk in one day.

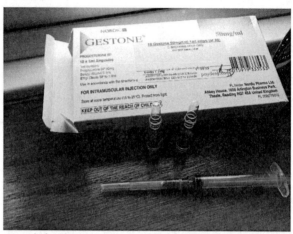

Gestone injections were prescribed to Verity in this cycle to assist in preventing miscarriage

10 weeks and 3 days pregnant:

I suffered slight dark brown bleed again Saturday night so instead of the one already booked for later this week (and mostly to calm our nerves) we are having a ten-week scan today. We've both been so incredibly nervous about it, I'm wondering if we should go ahead.

We are having it at our local hospital's early pregnancy unit. Although it's not the same one where we visited when we had one of the miscarriages, we're still suffering the fear of 'déjà vu'.

Post scan:

Being at the early pregnancy unit, this morning was horrible. The nerves were unbelievable! Pure fear.

When we arrived, we were in a tiny waiting room/corridor with about four other couples where you could hear everything that each of us were discussing. We were all in the same boat. You basically only visit here if something is potentially wrong. We were the last couple to go in and have a scan, and each couple came out happy bar one where we heard the poor lady saying to the nurse, "Sorry I'm crying…but yes if it's gone, it's gone." Paul and I looked at each other sadly for her and felt pure dread. We had been there ourselves. On the wall in front of us were posters about miscarriage, ectopic pregnancy and counselling. We were shaking.

Eventually, my name was called and we were taken through to a nurse. We had to fill in a massive form about our history (so it took a while)! She then said 'I won't do a pregnancy test as I'm sure everything's OK, but we usually do.' Then she changed her mind and said 'actually, maybe I should.' We were now worried. I did the test and we waited in the corridor again. Ten minutes later, she called us back. "Yes, it says you're still pregnant." Phew! However, from our past experiences we were very aware that you can of course have pregnancy hormones inside you for weeks if the worst has happened, so can have a positive pregnancy test (as I did previously).

After another 20 minutes or so, another door opened and another nurse called us in. This was it. The scan we'd be waiting for, but were oh so nervous about.

I lay on the bed and Paul and I held each other's clammy hands as the scanner went over my tummy; we wished each other 'good luck.'

Then, with a leap of joy in our hearts, we saw a little baby wriggling and dancing around inside of me. Our little miracle was there. The nurse then said, "Well, we are officially looking for a heartbeat but as you can see this little one is moving around perfectly." Relief filled our hearts…and love overflowed for this little being. Tears ran down our faces. She then printed us a picture and also pointed out to us the little heartbeat.

We then had to wait again, this time filled with joy and relief. Those posters couldn't upset us now. Nothing could.

Then the same door opened again, and the nurse said, "Verity, there's a slight problem; can you come back, please." *Oh no, what's happened?* We were worried once more. This is so typical of us, fine one minute then things can fall apart the next. Inside the room, she explained that she'd forgotten to measure my ovaries (which was needed as I had IVF apparently). Phew, that was all. So, lovely in a way, we were given a second viewing of our baby. What a wonderful day it had turned in to.

As we left the hospital, we somehow felt more pregnant! Happy, happy, happy!

Meanwhile, I am still injecting the Gestone each evening; or at least, poor Paul is.

A funny thing happened with the injections last week. I had run out of some of the needles. I was advised which chemist in Brighton near to us had those particular ones. So we visited. The pharmacist handed me a large brown paper bag full of all types of syringes, vitamin c and disinfectant towels (as we later discovered, these bags are usually intended for drug addicts). As they handed the bag to me over the counter the pharmacist said, "Carry it in a carrier bag as the police watch our chemist for drug dealers and they stop them. They may well stop you if they see you leaving here with one of our brown paper bags!" Paul and I ran to the car laughing all the way at the thought of being held up!

12 Week Scan:

Today was our 12-week scan to check that everything is developing, as it should be and also the first time that we were having a scan through the 'normal' procedures at our local NHS hospital where I would hopefully eventually give birth to this little being.

We were both nervous, and had suffered a few stressful workdays and were feeling anxious about this. Due to a big storm, we have also suffered a power cut at our house for the last 24 hours.

But here we were, on our way to hopefully see something great.

However, as soon as we stepped in to the hospital (literally on my first step inside the building over the threshold) I felt what I thought was a gush of water. Slightly alarmed with a sinking feeling, but not wanting to concern Paul, I told him that I needed the bathroom quickly. He didn't suspect anything luckily. He said there was a toilet in the scanning area, so I agreed to wait till we were in there. When we checked in at reception, I asked where the bathroom was and the receptionist informed me I could not go, as they needed me to have a full bladder for the scan. I said I had to 'wash my hands', and off I went to check what was going on.

Inside the bathroom, it was the one thing I dreaded as I looked down. I was bleeding. Bright red blood...and a lot of it!

I was shaking now with dread. I suddenly felt sick. This couldn't be happening. Not when we'd come this far.

I came out to Paul, he looked at my face as I stepped out towards him in the waiting area and he said with fear, "What is it, what's wrong?" I just nodded and although I then gently informed him, I also played it down so as not to worry him too much. I just said there was some 'slight red discharge, a bit more than previously'.

The shock was great enough for me, why put him through that too! If something bad had happened, I wanted to at least let him down slowly. I wanted to protect him.

We sat waiting for the scan, feeling sick. I couldn't stop shaking. It felt like forever.

When we were called through, I quickly informed the sonographer lady what had happened. She immediately took control getting everything prepared for the scan quickly. As I lay on the bed and the scan began, we both tried eagerly to see our baby on the screen. I could feel tears running down my face. She quickly said, "Well, there is your baby!" We braced ourselves for the heartbeat news. "And there is its heartbeat flickering away!" Oh my goodness, the relief was amazing. We had entered the room not knowing what to expect…but here we were seeing our beloved baby moving and apparently even 'sucking its thumb or fingers' already. It had its legs crossed and then moved around wriggling. We were overjoyed, but also in shock from the last few minutes' events. And what was that sudden bleeding?

She measured everything and all looked perfect. Then she started to look around my tummy for the reason for the bleed. The only significant thing she could find was that the placenta was lying low. It should ideally be to the side. Apparently, this can sometimes cause bleeding.

Afterwards, we went to see the midwife who took my necessary bloods and explained the whole meaning of a low-lying placenta. At our next scan, 20 weeks, it should hopefully have shifted to one the side as the uterus would have grown more by then. In most cases, it does apparently. Worst-case scenario, and it doesn't, I would just need a caesarean. After what I've gone through to get to this stage, that's absolutely nothing.

We are also booked to see the obstetrician next week as I'm under the 'special care' category. So I am sure we will discuss it all in more detail then.

In the meantime, we are at home now under candle light with still no electricity. But I am bleeding still on and off which is very scary. Perhaps, it is a good thing that I can't Google anything tonight (with no WiFi).

What a roller coaster this continues to be. But how amazing it has been today seeing our beautiful baby sucking fingers and moving around. We've decided not to tell anyone about our worrying episode today, as not to worry our families or to make more of a big deal of it to us. We will just keep it to ourselves.

I am going to rest a bit more from now on though until everything settles.

13 Weeks Pregnant, Into 2nd Trimester:

I'd forgotten that with our due date being moved forward slightly, that I was now in the second trimester yesterday. When I discovered this (on a pregnancy app I use), I was on cloud nine! This is another amazing milestone for us. It makes me gradually feel *normal*.

Thankfully, the heavy bleeding stopped the day after it started.

Our pregnancy is also public knowledge now, which is so lovely. Even though, we are still telling people that we are cautious.

So, Wednesday we are meeting our obstetrician. We are going to request another scan, just because from now until 20 weeks seems a long way off.

It's so rewarding seeing Niomi and my parents so excited now as time goes by; all of us are starting to relax day by day. Everyone is guessing the sex now! I still can't believe this is happening. Currently, Paul and I think a boy. My mother thinks a boy as does Paul's stepfather, John, and the majority of our close friends. Although, Niomi thinks it is a girl. We've decided not to find out the sex and go down the old-fashioned, traditional route – we simply think that for us, after all we've been through, the idea of being handed our baby when it's born and being told 'congratulations it's a…' is a moment we've always dreamt about together. We also feel we've had enough help using modern techniques. For us, we will be happy with whatever we are blessed with. A healthy baby really is all we pray for.

13 Weeks 6 Days Pregnant:

Yesterday, we met with the obstetrician at our hospital. I must say, we went in to the meeting feeling happy as the midwife who had just taken my blood pressure asked if we would like to hear the baby's heartbeat, which of course we did. Paul was especially surprised at how fast the little heartbeat was. It all came flooding back to me from when I had Niomi. We were both elated! The nurse told us it was a good strong heartbeat. So happy.

However, upon meeting the obstetrician, he was immediately negative, in a flap with paper work and hard to understand as he kept muttering under his breath to himself. Very odd.

He told us in great detail about preeclampsia (even though I have very low blood pressure and am only 13 weeks pregnant). And then, all about if I catch a cold while coming off my prednisolone (which I told him I am gradually reducing as instructed by The Lister Hospital) I could end up in intensive care! He also thought all the drugs that fertility clinics give patients should be tried against the placebo effect. In other words, he didn't 'believe in IVF'. He didn't say one positive thing or smile at us...not even slightly. The trouble is I'm an optimist, and so, I just didn't gel with him at all.

Fortunately, one of my best friends whose sister is a local GP has recommended an obstetrician we should request from now on. I'm calling the hospital tomorrow.

Meanwhile, after days of nothing, I had some more slight bleeding again this morning. It has stopped since, but still I will keep an eye on it. It's very stressful! And have had a bad headache all day.

16 Weeks Pregnant:

I've had a lovely slight fluttering in my tummy over the last week on and off which could be the baby moving. It's amazing! I can't wait for Paul to be able to feel his baby too.

I was also naughty and went on to Amazon and bought a handheld Doppler to hear the baby's heartbeat at home. We thought we wouldn't get one in case it caused anxiety. However, in actual fact it's calmed any anxieties that I especially have due to the bleed. It's amazing too. And Niomi has been able to hear her baby sibling, which is lovely to see.

17 Weeks:

After the slight fluttering, just as I was 17 weeks 3 days, I felt some proper big kicks so I quickly called Paul. He placed his hand on my belly…nothing. I kept saying, "There, did you feel it?" Nothing.

He looked quite sad so I felt bad. Then suddenly a big kick or movement happened and he said with an enormous grin and tears in his eyes, "Yes, there it is. I felt it!"

It was such an amazing moment for us both…one that at times we questioned if we would ever share.

18 Weeks:

The baby is now moving a lot more, mostly evenings and when I get in to bed. Although, this morning I did feel a big prod pushing outwards as if the baby was saying 'get up mummy, I need breakfast in you'! Paul also felt this big movement. Hugely happy days!

We are having an extensive scan in Harley Street tomorrow that one of my best friends had with her two babies that looks at every organ of the baby in great detail. We are doing everything to be cautious after all we've been through.

20 Weeks Today:

Our scan in London was incredible and now back home we keep looking at the images and DVD.

The baby is kicking so much – even as I write this! Paul loves feeling it too. It's just amazing.

I can't believe we've made it to the halfway mark! We are both so elated. We are also relaxing more with each day that passes. After all these years of hope, pain and despair, it's still sinking in that we are getting there and that we are expecting a baby!

We held a Christmas party at our home last week which was so lovely (showed off the bump) and in five days it is Christmas Day (we are having some of our family over and I am cooking 12 of us). It's such a positive exciting time.

Nearly 21 weeks, Christmas Day today:

Christmas Day is here! So far, it's been an eventful run up to it. We are entertaining ten family members for dinner today and late last night Paul, Niomi and I discovered we had no water just before we went to bed! It's due to another terrible storm that occurred last night. We also had the loudest bolt of thunder we've ever heard. And so I didn't sleep as a result between 3–7 a.m. Fortunately, our water was back on when we got up this morning. But needless to say, I am now feeling tired. I'm looking forward to today though. And as I type this lying down, the baby is kicking frantically. First Christmas for bump!

22 Weeks and 2 Days:

On Boxing Day, we had our NHS 22 week scan. The baby was absolutely fine and beautiful. But the sonographer found some tiny specks of blood in the amniotic fluid surrounding the baby. She has assured us it is nothing to worry about and that there is no sign of any bleeding, but naturally, we do worry! She referred us to the on-duty doctor there who also reassured us but requested we return for another scan at 24 weeks. So we are booked in. She also asked me to just keep an eye on the movements of the baby each day and that if I become concerned to call them.

Meanwhile I'd had numerous blood tests done at my GP's surgery checking my iron and thyroid levels, so when I called for the results I spoke to my GP who also assured me not to worry about the specks of blood and said it wouldn't affect the baby. Phew. In fact, babies can apparently healthily swallow it.

Meanwhile, last night I noticed the baby hadn't moved for a while. Anyway, I managed to worry myself and stayed awake most of the night as a result! Then today I felt only minor flutters so still worried a bit. Paul and I listened to the heartbeat on our monitor so you'd think I would feel reassured. But it sounded different, so I worried that was the flow of the placenta pulsing that you can apparently sometimes hear instead of the heartbeat.

Anyway, this evening sitting on the sofa as I am now I am elated to say that baby is back to its kicking little self again! A big relief for over-anxious mummy (and daddy).

Looking back, I think it had moved position in to my lower pelvis, as I've been to the toilet a lot more than usual. So it was pushing on my bladder.

I'm sitting here happy now with Paul and Niomi looking and feeling the kicks.

We've also had more business stresses this week (as usually happens when you own your own business) so I was worried it had affected the baby.

22 Weeks and 6 Days:

Had my first pregnant swim today. Due to our earlier complications with the bleed and then the placenta praevia (low lying placenta) I was told I couldn't swim.

So having been told I can now swim, I really enjoyed it so much! And it helped with some rib and back pain that I have suffered lately.

24 Weeks and 2 Days:

Feel amazing to be reaching each of these milestones.

Last week we looked at prams, which was so exciting. And although some people say it's still too early for us after all we've been through, we find it actually helps to be focusing on positivity. After all, that's what's got us through these six years!

The other day we had someone telling me in great detail about a miscarriage they had a while back. As distressing as that clearly was for them (and we know only too well), we see it as unhealthy to dwell and focus on such things (especially as they subsequently have had more children easily, naturally). We find it better to focus on good positive stories; that's just our way. I feel as though I have moved on from the miscarriages and ectopic. Whatever life throws at you, it's better for yourself to surely only carry the good baggage with you and leave the rest behind. I will always have pain in my heart of course from those experiences. But I must move on now.

25 Weeks:

Yesterday we had the scan that the hospital requested as the previous one showed specks of blood in the amniotic fluid.

Thankfully, the specks had decreased to only a few blood clots that the doctor said were absolutely not harmful at all and are fine now. We asked again if they could harm the baby if swallowed and she reassured us they couldn't at all. It's another little hurdle that we are over. The doctor also commented how the placenta has continued moving up and is in the perfect position now.

So, we saw our gorgeous little miracle kicking and moving around once again. The sonographer told us how our little one now has fat deposits on its cheeks and chin, and weighs a pound and a half. So happy and relieved.

The funny thing is that we went into this scan both feeling calm. Perhaps we sensed all might be fine this time as the baby is kicking so much.

I'm growing a lot now too (although Paul says I still don't look pregnant anywhere other than the bump! He says it's like a torpedo at the front of me. One of my best friends says it's like I have a football under my top). I love seeing my bump and showing it off. Being pregnant is something all pregnant women should be proud of. I feel very well too. I am still just getting tired in the afternoons and still have this rib/diaphragm/back pain quite often. And most nights, I wake up yelling with a sudden cramp in my foot or toes in spasm. Poor Paul gets quite a shock when I scream!

Other than these minor ailments (that I'm so happy to be in a position of having) the bruises on my buttocks where the Gestone injections were (I've stopped thankfully now) still hurt. I think it's the nerves under the muscle. For example, last night in bed I had a sharp deep pain from one of the bumps in my buttocks shooting down to my toes. It's all worth it though. And yes of course I'd do it all again. We still keep saying every day that we can't believe we are in this privileged position.

25 Weeks and 1 Day:

After having a few weeks of having my energy back again, I've noticed that in the last few days I'm feeling ever so tired most of the time. I suspect it's something to do with me now approaching the third trimester. I'm also on iron tablets for anaemia, so maybe that's why (it flagged up in a routine blood test that my iron levels are just slightly under). Anyway, I am seeing the midwife in two days' time so I will mention it then. Also, being a sufferer of low blood pressure, it could be that. But hey ho, all is good and I am so happy.

I must say, that throughout this pregnancy so far, kind words, cards and gifts that my friends have been giving me have overwhelmed me. My close-knit friends, I now know, really did feel and see the pain I was going through all these years; it makes me feel guilty that they worried so. I am very lucky to have such special friends in my life. From relaxing bath oils to plaques about friendship and cards of 'happy congratulations' with heartfelt words; I feel truly blessed.

Over the Christmas period, I sent Raef Faris a card and informed him how well we are doing (thanks to him and his team)! I also told him how we look forward to the day when we take our little one to visit everybody at The Lister Hospital! That makes me smile so much.

28 Weeks and 4 Days:

I've just been to visit the midwife at our GP's surgery for a general checkup. The baby's heartbeat is perfect and the uterus is 28 cm which is also perfect (it should measure the amount of weeks pregnant in centimetres).

I informed the midwife how since around eight weeks pregnant I've been suffering bad deep pain under my left front ribs; in the diaphragm area. It seems to be getting a lot worse when I sit or drive. She said it was probably a pulled muscle but then mentioned that, "It could of course be a small fracture in a rib from coughing or sneezing without realising it." I can take paracetamol, but I've avoided it so far. Though if it gets much worse, I might try just one. As I write this, it is very painful now.

However, I am willing to go through anything to be at this happy stage and refuse to grumble.

I must say that apart from the rib pain, I really am enjoying this pregnancy so much (unsurprisingly). I'm now well and truly in the third trimester and am still feeling great. My friends keep saying how much pregnancy suits me too; I think it is pure happiness to be in this position. It is a remarkable feeling and both Paul and I still have to keep pinching ourselves that this is actually happening. I guess we always will. So blessed, so happy.

I am doing the Lucozade blood test at the end of this week (it measures sugar in your blood an hour after drinking a small bottle of Lucozade. Great marketing for the drinks brand)!

31 Weeks:

I had to go back to have the glucose 'Lucozade' test done again as my levels were very slightly elevated.

Had to get to the hospital early in the morning with an empty stomach (which never agrees with me, giving me the shakes).

I had to drink a solution when I got there this time and then stay on the premises for two hours. Got very bored. But then, I suddenly got faint when sitting on a chair towards the end of the two-hour wait. I was alone. I managed to stay seated when this happened, no one noticed thankfully. I then went outside for some fresh air which made me feel much better.

I then sat watching couples departing the hospital with their new babies in little car seats. I kept picturing us doing that.

Anyway, I've now had the results and thankfully all is OK, within the perfect range now. They think it was because I ate lots of cake the day before the original test! Typical me, loving my cake.

35 Weeks:

I have been suffering with this diaphragm pain on my left side for months now, and I've been seeing my chiropractor about it which does help.

However, this week it seems to have subsided which is great. And in addition, people have commented that the bump has dropped lower. I had a wonderful surprise baby shower this week organised by Niomi and my mother. It was great fun, and quite emotional for me, especially when I did a small 'thank you for being here' speech to my friends and family. It was one of those surreal moments when it suddenly hit me as I stood there in front of everyone that I am actually really pregnant. And there I was sharing this amazing moment in my life with people I love. Niomi organised some great games. We played one where everyone had to guess the baby's sex. Most were saying 'girl', and I must say I have been thinking for some time now that it's a girl, and so is Paul. But who knows…

So, since everyone says the bump is now lower, I am wondering if the baby is engaging?

My chiropractor did also say that when the baby engages the pain should go.

However, at our previous scan two weeks ago (the hospital requested it due to the specks of blood in the amniotic fluid), the baby was in the breech position. It has been moving a lot more lately though so I am wondering if it has now turned.

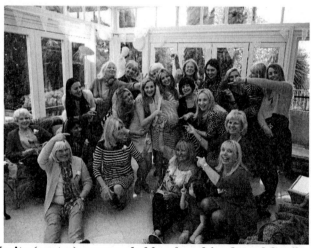

Verity (centre) surrounded by close friends and family at her baby shower

38 Weeks:

I saw the midwife two weeks ago, who informed me that the baby has indeed engaged (3/5 of the way) and that she most probably wouldn't see me two weeks later as she suspected I may have the baby before that.

However, here I am awaiting for my appointment to see her this afternoon.

Today I woke up feeling sick and generally not my usual self. And throughout another sleepless night, I felt dizzy even in bed (despite lying on my side).

So, now Paul and I are wondering if this could be the beginning...very excited and of course apprehensive...but can't wait to meet our little miracle.

39 Weeks:

Five days before my due date, in the early hours of bank holiday Monday 5th May, I started to get cramping feelings.

I thought I'd let Paul sleep on as I had a sneaky suspicion I'd need his full energy as my coach that day! Once the cramps became strong, I woke him and we decided to make 'that telephone call' to the hospital.

They advised we pop up there for a check. As I walked to the bathroom I had a 'show'. This really was happening now!

At the hospital, they checked the baby's heartbeat and examined me and decided I was in labour. However, I was OK to go home for a few hours.

In between, at about 7 a.m., Paul and I took a walk around the grounds of the hospital. It was a beautiful sunny May morning, peaceful (as no one was there, it being a bank holiday) and we were both surprisingly extremely relaxed and calm. I called Niomi to notify her and my mother of what was now happening, gently. Paul and I sat on a bench enjoying the morning sun and simply listened to the birds singing as we held hands; it couldn't have begun more beautifully.

Then, we departed home to go to bed for a few hours (as advised by the midwife).

However, just as I climbed in to bed, I felt my waters break! OK, I knew this could be fast (if anything like my daughter Niomi's birth which was about one hour) so I called the hospital.

163

The midwife simply said, "You need to get here quick and now! Do you want an ambulance sent to you?" I said we would be fine, as I knew living where we are in the Sussex countryside; it would be quicker for us to leave by car immediately. I called to Paul who had gone downstairs…very oddly, he was putting a pie in the oven! Very out of character. Looking back, he says he doesn't know why he did it, and that he just thought, *right, we need to eat before we leave since the midwife had informed us that giving birth is like running a marathon, so we'd need energy*! He's a strategic person so I think he felt he had to do something practical (and caring too). Something I am sure I will always tease him about.

We quickly gathered everything I needed and off we went…to finally have our miracle baby.

5ᵗʰ May 2014:

At 2:40 p.m., after the most incredibly natural happy birth the baby that we had so longed for so many years finally made her appearance in to the big wide world. Our little Daisy-May arrived after a very quick and relatively easy birth. Love filled our hearts for her from the moment we could see her little body for the very first time. It was a quick, non-complicated and almost spiritual birth; calm surrounded the room throughout.

I was placed in a private room and for the whole of her first night at the hospital with me, I simply sat watching every inch of her and every breath that she took. I was overflowing with love. Will this little being ever know how much she was wanted by us? We will make sure she does. For we will shower this little girl with love for the whole of her life.

Now as we look back upon this turbulent journey over the past 6 years, we ask ourselves "What led our dream to become a reality on this final cycle?"

There are many various factors, and so we come to the conclusion that it was the perfect storm of all of them together.

From the relaxing holiday in Lake Como prior to this cycle to the Gestone injections to the hysteroscopy and endometrial scratching…or had some fertility luck of sitting next to Professor Robert Winston on the beach in Lake Como rubbed off on to me? Or was it simply that we went in to this cycle feeling blasé that this was our final chance? In a way, we felt the pressure had dispersed since we had almost conceded that it wasn't going to work.

We will never know, but I had to simply keep these notes and write this book in the hope that it might help others. If it can help even one couple by pointing them in the right direction of what techniques to try or where to go, or it simply gives someone emotional support when they are on their fertility journey, then I have achieved all that I wanted to with this book.

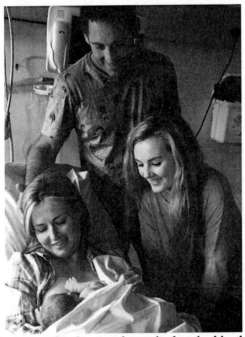

Daisy-May soon after her much-awaited arrival in the arms of Verity, with Paul and big sister Niomi (right)

At 8 weeks old, we took Daisy-May for a very special visit. A journey to meet the wonderful team at The Lister Hospital who made her arrival possible. Our visit was not only for them to meet Daisy-May, but also an opportunity for us to thank them. It was emotional. I was extremely hot. I don't know whether that was the warm weather or my emotions; I'd guess the latter.

We took flowers, chocolates and cards for the team, which to us seemed so lame. But how do you thank people for what we now have and for such kindness shown to us over the years? It's a strange situation because some of them, in particular such as Raef and Safira, had become in a sense friends of ours; they knew more than people close to us what we were going through and they helped us not just physiologically but also emotionally. We know that they went over and above protocol; but as they used to tell us, our case was an unusual one.

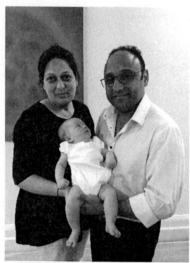

Safira Batha (head of embryology) and Raef Faris at The Lister Hospital with Daisy-May

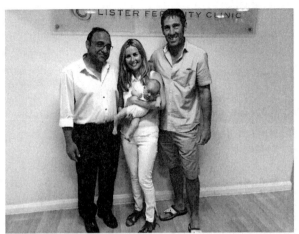

When Daisy-May was two months old, Verity and Paul took her to meet Raef Faris (their consultant at The Lister)

We will miss them. But one thing we shall always make sure of is that as Daisy-May grows up she will know all about them.

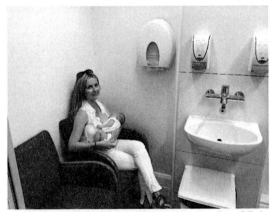

Verity proudly feeding Daisy-May (two months old) in one of the consulting rooms at The Lister where she would have previously experienced many difficult medical discussions about the couple's struggle to have a baby

A year later after the birth of our dear little Daisy-May, we held her christening at our house in the garden beside our pond. It was naturally a very moving and emotional day, one that we had always dreamt of and that we will treasure forever. But it was made even more special as we had invited Raef Faris to join us, and he did. Having him there, introducing him to our parents and Niomi, was a true privilege for us and for them to be able to also thank him for our beautiful new addition in our family; there were tears from us all as we chatted to him. Paul did a speech and informed our guests that we had 'a true VIP amongst us today'.

So dreams and miracles can come true…and we are proof. After all, we were told by two fertility doctors that we would never have a baby of our own together. Thankfully, Mr Raef Faris and Dr Michael Dooley believed otherwise! And so did our hearts.

So, our message to anyone going through a similar journey to ours now? Firstly, we genuinely think of you every day.

Secondly, if you have the mental strength (and finances to do so), don't give up if your heart is telling you to keep going. I am a true believer in listening to your personal instinct.

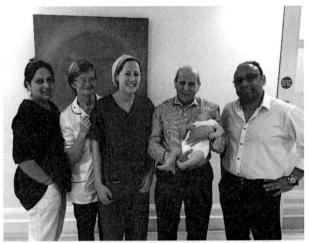

'The wonderful team' at The Lister Hospital meet Daisy-May for the first time (From left – Safira Batha, head of embryology, Alison, one of the sonographers, Katherine, from the embryology department, and consultants Mr Mahmoud Tolba, holding Daisy-May, and Mr Raef Faris)